Essential Skills Clusters for Nurses

Essential Skills Clusters for Nurses
Theory for Practice

Edited by

Linda Louise Childs
MSc, BSc (Hons), RN, RHV, DNcert, NP,
PG Dip (Nurse Education) RNT, Fellow HEA
University of Southampton

Lesley Coles
BA, RN, DN, RM, RHV, RNT, Cert Ed, Fellow HEA
University of Southampton

and

Barbara Marjoram
TD, MA, RN, Cert Ed, Fellow HEA
University of Southampton

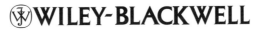

WILEY-BLACKWELL
A John Wiley & Sons, Ltd., Publication

This edition first published 2009
© 2009 by Blackwell Publishing Ltd

Blackwell Publishing was acquired by John Wiley & Sons in February 2007.
Blackwell's publishing programme has been merged with Wiley's global Scientific, Technical, and Medical
business to form Wiley-Blackwell.

Registered office
John Wiley & Sons Ltd, The Atrium, Southern Gate, Chichester, West Sussex,
PO19 8SQ, United Kingdom

Editorial offices
9600 Garsington Road, Oxford, OX4 2DQ, United Kingdom
2121 State Avenue, Ames, Iowa 50014-8300, USA

For details of our global editorial offices, for customer services and for information about how to apply
for permission to reuse the copyright material in this book please see our website at www.wiley.com/wiley-
blackwell.

Library of Congress Cataloging-in-Publication Data
Essential skills clusters for nurses : theory for practice / edited by Linda
Louise Childs, Lesley Coles, Barbara Marjoram.
    p. ; cm.
  Includes bibliographical references and index.
  ISBN 978-1-4051-8341-3 (pbk. : alk. paper) 1. Nursing. I. Childs, Linda
  Louise. II. Coles, Lesley. III. Marjoram, Barbara A.
  [DNLM: 1. Nursing Care—methods. 2. Nurse-Patient Relations. 3. Nursing
  Care—organization & administration. WY 100 E783 2009]
    RT41.E86 2009
    610.73—dc22

                                                  2008039847

A catalogue record for this book is available from the British Library.

Set in 10/12 pt Sabon by Newgen Imaging Systems (P) Ltd, Chennai, India
Printed and bound in Malaysia by Vivar Printing Sdn Bhd

1   2009

Contents

Foreword

As someone whose professional responsibilities centre around professional education policy, I am delighted to have been invited to write the foreword to this book that aims to provide the theoretical underpinning for Essential Nursing Skills and thereby provide the essential understanding for safe and effective practice. Its publication is timely as it coincides with the introduction of the Nursing and Midwifery Council's (NMC) Essential Skills Clusters for pre-registration nursing education required to be introduced from September 2008.

The NMC is the UK regulator for two professions, nursing and midwifery. The primary purpose of the NMC is to safeguard the health and well-being of the public. It does this through setting standards for the education, training, conduct and for entry to the nursing and midwifery register within the United Kingdom and by maintaining a register of all nurses and midwives who meet the requirements of fitness to practice (currently more than 674 000 nurses and midwives are registered).

So just where did the Essential Skills Clusters come from and why, and how significant is their introduction? In 2005, the NMC consulted on a number of practice-related issues around fitness for practice at the point of registration. I was privileged to have been close to the action and to see what led ultimately to the development of Essential Skills Clusters for pre-registration nursing and the issuing of NMC Circular 07/2007.

Back in 2005 there were suggestions that some newly registered nurses might not be as competent as they might be at the point of registration. The NMC decided to act by setting out a number of proposals for consultation, including how to better support students' learning in practice, how to strengthen assessment of practice learning and how to more effectively support the achievement of existing NMC outcomes and proficiencies for pre-registration nursing education in some skill areas.

The consultation subsequently led to the development of five generic Essential Skills Clusters. Aided by experts from each field, and drawing on an evidence base, Essential Skills Clusters were developed for, care, compassion and communication, organisational aspects of care, infection prevention and control, nutrition and fluid management and medicines management. These Essential Skills Clusters will be evaluated once they have become established and may evolve according to need and the future frameworks for pre-registration nurse education.

Developing the Essential Skills Clusters was about ensuring safe and effective practice, and making valid and reliable judgements. It was also about practice competence and maintaining the public's safety, trust and confidence, principles that are strengthened through the evidence base underpinning essential skills as developed in this text. This book identifies the theory which underpins these Essential Skills Clusters to support the development of best nursing practice. I hope you enjoy it.

Garth Long,
Professional Advisor,
Education, Nursing and Midwifery Council

List of Contributors

Palo Almond PhD, MSc, PG Dip Ed, PG Dip AHCP, BSc (Hons), Dip HV, RM, RGN, RNT, University of Southampton

Robert Henry Carter BA (Hons), PG Dip HRM, MSc, University of Southampton

Linda Louise Childs MSc, BSc (Hons), RN, RHV, DNcert, NP, PG Dip (Nurse Education) RNT, Fellow HEA, University of Southampton

Joan Cochrane MSc (Health), RN, RM, DNcert, Northumbria University

Michelle Denise Cowen MSc (SpLD), RN, BEd (Hons), University of Southampton

Sue M. Green RN, BSc, MMedSci, PhD, PG Cert, University of Southampton

Kevin Humphrys RN, MSc (Applied Psychology), Cert Ed (FE), University of Southampton

Paula Libberton BN (Hons) (Mental Health), RN, PG Dip (Education), University of Southampton

Garth Long RN (Adult), RN (Mental Health), MA (Ed), BEd, DipN, PGCE, Professional Advisor, Education, Nursing and Midwifery Council

Jane Caroline Portlock BPharm (Hons), MRPharmS, PhD, FHEA, University of Portsmouth

Beth Sepion RSCN, RGN, SCM, BEd (Hons), MSc, University of Southampton

Carmel Sheppard RGN, BSc (Hons), MSc, DBMS, Dip Counselling, Portsmouth Hospital Trust

Jane Smith RNLD, Diploma Nursing Sciences, Hampshire Partnership Trust

Cathy Sullivan RN, MSc, University of Southampton

Stephen Richard Tee DClinP, PGCEA, MA, BA (Hons), DPSN, RMN, University of Southampton

Pauline Turner BA (Hons), MPhil, RN, Diploma Palliative Care, University of Southampton

Wendy Wigley EN (G), RN, Dip HE (Child health), BSc (Hons) (Community Care), PG Cert (Education), University of Southampton

Lyn Wilson BSc, PGCE, MSc, University of Southampton

Jackie Yardley MA (Ed), RN, RHV, Diploma in Counselling, Master Practitioner NLP, EHPNLP, PG Dip (Applied Clinical Hypnosis), Cert CBT, University of Southampton

List of Tables

List of Figures

List of Boxes

Introduction

This text is designed to be used as a study guide to support the theoretical aspects of the Nursing and Midwifery Council's (NMC 2007) Essential Skills Clusters that were introduced as compulsory elements, from 2008, to pre-registration nursing programmes. Students on other programmes may also find the text very useful, for example, those undertaking the Return to Practice, Foundation Degree programmes.

Each chapter has been written by subject specialists and we hope that their enthusiasm for their topic areas is evident when you read them. The chapters are not designed to be read in any particular order and should be tackled when you feel they are relevant to your learning. The learning outcomes give you an idea of what you can achieve when you are working through the chapters.

The book is divided into five sections. Each section discusses a particular area of the Essential Skills Clusters. Section 1 explores care, compassion and communication and includes a chapter on communication with related chapters exploring communicating in various settings. Although not designed to cover all aspects of communication this section discusses areas of care that affect this important topic.

Section 2 explores organisational aspects of care and includes chapters on management, promoting health and well-being, legal and ethical aspects of health care.

Section 3 explores infection prevention and control.

Section 4 explores nutrition and fluid management.

Section 5 explores medicines management and the pharmacology.

The cross-referencing, between each chapter, increases the coherence of the text. Activities have been included, in each chapter, to help you develop insights into the areas being discussed and your own practice/learning.

Reference

Nursing and Midwifery Council (NMC) (2007) Essential Skills Clusters. NMC Circular 07(2007) Annexe 2, NMC, London.

Section 1

Care, Compassion and Communication

CHAPTER 1

An Introduction to Communication

Palo Almond and Jackie Yardley

Introduction

There is an abundance of literature on communication which is seen as central to quality health care services and is identified as an essential skill (NMC 2007b); and yet the skills of communication remain lacking within the health care professions and every year complaints in the National Health Service (NHS) continue to be focused on misunderstanding based on poor communication (Pincock 2004).

Not all problems are communication problems, however; a skilled communicator can facilitate meaning and understanding in a given situation bringing clarity to an issue that otherwise would escalate out of control. Part of the difficulty lies in the fact that we communicate all the time and for most this is an activity that is valued and almost everyone agrees is important; but this chapter is asking you to consider your communication skills as if for the first time and reflect on where change would enable you to employ the principles and process of a skilled communicator.

This chapter is divided into three sections. The first section focuses on some of the policy imperatives that require nurses to ensure that they have the knowledge and skills to communicate with all people whatever their age, gender, disability, sexual orientation or ethnicity might be. The second section places communication skills centre stage within health care and therapeutic settings and explores what it means to communicate. Finally, the third section explores some of the evidence base currently influencing communication and delivery of health care.

The specific learning outcomes addressed in this chapter link with the Nursing and Midwifery Council's (NMC 2007b) Essential Skills Clusters, and are identified below.

Learning outcomes

By the end of this chapter you will be able to do the following:

- Identify the term health inequality and recognise how communication is an important factor in accessing health care.
- Describe the importance of policy and how it aims to reduce health inequalities.
- Establish different theoretical perspectives increasing your understanding of communication.
- Identify the key principles of effective communication so that appropriate communication strategies can be employed.
- Examine the importance of self-awareness and how attitudes, beliefs and values can create barriers to effective communication.
- Explain how effective communication can enhance practice.
- Use a case study approach to explore evidence-based, ethically and culturally sensitive communication practice.

Inequalities in Health: Provision and Access to Health Care

Many sectors of society are at risk of having poor health due to difficulties in access to health care or because health care does not meet the specific needs of all groups in mind. It is beyond the scope of this chapter to appraise all barriers to health care faced by service users including ethnic minority populations residing in the United Kingdom. Instead, this chapter focuses on a specific barrier that many patients face, that is effective two-way communication. Robinson (2002) appraised 134 studies related to communication and provides evidence of the part that communication plays in creating barriers to providing quality health care or accessing health care by patients who do not have English as their first language. However, it needs to be stated at the outset that not all patients experience difficulties in communication and not all minority ethnic patients are not fluent in communicating in written or oral English. Indeed, many patients are very satisfied with the care they receive. In this chapter, the term patient is used instead of the more cumbersome 'patients or clients'. It is accepted that either of the two terms can be applied in most health care settings. The focal point of this chapter is on access issues relating to communication with minority ethnic patients, when the ethnicity of the patient is different to that of the nurse. The final section discusses some of the barriers to effective communication that may cause inequality in access and how these might be avoided.

The Black Report (Townsend & Davidson 1982) and *The Health Divide* (Whitehead 1988)

Both these studies found marked differences in the health of certain sections of the UK population. The researchers theorised that these differences were preventable by addressing the provision and delivery of health services and other public services. Such changes would increase access by those who need health and social services. Governments of that time appeared not to have taken any policy actions to address these reported health inequalities. Their ideology emphasised less Government control over people's health, and greater responsibility by individuals for their own health (Baggott 2000; Ham 2004). Ten years later, Acheson (1998) found that the gap between the health of the well off and the less well off was as wide or wider. An analysis of policy in the last 10 years suggests a more positive attitude to the need to reduce and prevent health inequalities.

Government Health Policy and Legislation

Analysis of policy suggests that some formal steps have been attempted to reduce health inequalities in the United Kingdom. *Saving Lives: Our Healthier Nation* (Department of Health (DH) 1998) set out,

> ... to improve the health of the worst off in society at a faster rate than the rest of the population. (DH 1998, p. 1)

This reflects a willingness to accept that inequalities do exist, and that Government action needs to be taken. Consequently, the Government set targets to reduce inequalities in *The NHS Plan* (DH 2000). The Government noted causative structural factors and particular populations most at risk of poorer health:

> The social and economic determinants of health remain important factors. Poverty, ethnic origin, and low educational achievement are all potentially significant issues. The determinants of health give rise to inequalities in health between different socio-economic and ethnic groups. (*The NHS Improvement Plan: A Plan for Investment, a Plan for Reform*, DH 2004a, p. 43)

This policy emphasised that people experiencing social and economic adversity and minority ethnic populations have less good health than other sectors of the population and that this situation is avoidable and needs addressing. The *National Service Framework for Children, Young People, and Maternity Services* (DH 2004b) also emphasises that the needs of people, who may have difficulties in accessing health services should be met by tailoring services that best meet their requirements. The predecessor to *The NHS Improvement Plan: A Plan for Investment, a Plan for Reform* (DH 2004a), *The NHS Plan* (DH 2000), was the very first UK policy to set targets for the reduction of health inequalities.

Chapter 3 of the *Equality Act* (2006) discusses equality and human rights and diversity. The main purpose of the Act is to set out the powers of the new Commission for Equality and Human Rights. Nevertheless, the Act raises awareness of the points made earlier that difference, that is ethnic diversity, should be acknowledged and not ignored. This builds on the 2000 *Race Relations (Amendment) Act* which set out the statutory responsibilities of health and local authorities to examine discriminatory practices and promote equality. Health services have a duty to provide culturally sensitive services (*Race Relations Amendment Act* 2000) (Activity 1.1).

> **Activity 1.1**
>
> To learn more about the Human Rights Act 1998 (HRA98) you could read the section on *Human Rights Act* 1998 (HRA98) in Chapter 9 of this book.

Policy Guiding Health Care Practice

The Government have clearly been aware that health inequalities can arise from poorly trained staff who are not competent and do not provide appropriate and accessible care. Consequently, the Government have taken action and set benchmarks for best health care practice, in the form of *Essence of Care* (DH 2001). It recommends that nurses and other health and social care professionals need to consider,

> Patients and or carers' individual needs or special needs including ethnicity, religion, culture, language, age, physical, sensory, developmental and psychological requirements. (DH 2001, p. 12)

A specific benchmark has been set for communication between health professionals and between the health professional and the patient. For instance, it states that

> patients and carers experience effective communication, sensitive to their individual needs and preferences, that promotes high quality care for the patient. (DH NHS Modernisation Agency 2003, p. 1)

Additionally, the *Essential Skills Clusters for Pre-Registration Nursing Programmes* (NMC 2007b) includes a key requirement of all newly registered nurses to have the ability to treat patients with dignity and respect them as individuals. The *Care, Compassion, and Communication* skills cluster requires nurses to respect diversity, be culturally competent, be non-discriminatory and not to harass or exploit patients. Nurses should be able to demonstrate an understanding of how culture, religion, spiritual beliefs, gender and sexuality can impact on illness and disability (NMC 2007b, p. 5). Nurses are therefore required to promote care that is sensitive to patient differences. Cultural competent practice can be defined as,

> A requirement of a practitioner to have culturally relevant knowledge, skills, and attitudes when working with diverse populations. To have an attitude of respect and openness to learn and provide effective health care which takes account of people's cultural beliefs, needs and behaviours. (Almond 2008, p. 229)

Effective communication is also reliant on the nurse working in partnership with patients. Almond and Cowley (2008) provide a skills typology for working in partnership with patients and clients. It is founded on egalitarian and ethical principles. To work in this way the nurse requires a moral framework, to help her practice ethically and sensitively. Such a framework involves developing an understanding that all patients have a right to good quality health care, all patients

---

Activity 1.2

Think of two people that you consider as excellent communicators and observe how they interact with people. What do they 'do' that makes them excellent at communication? Can you adopt these actions to improve your communication skills?

---

should be enabled to access the care provided and that barriers are removed for patients to access health care. These barriers are not concerned with geographical or physical barriers but are more often related to difficulties in communication (Gerrish *et al.* 1996).

This overview provides the policy drivers for nurses' communication practice. It is argued that if health inequalities are to be prevented, nurses need to develop and practice communication skills that do not exclude patients and prevent them from getting the care they have a right to. The chapter now presents some of the general theories of communication, but it may be helpful to undertake Activity 1.2 before reading further.

What is Communication?

Communication is a process of interaction, meaning and understanding, in other words a message is passed from one individual to the intended individual and/or group of people and will be received or not, interpreted or not, understood and/or misunderstood. The message can also act as a trigger creating a positive or negative response which in turn can affect the responding message and behaviour of the individual and/or group. Consider also in this process that other factors influence the message and response of any given individual that when you enter these factors into the context of the situation you begin to understand the complexities of communication.

Communication is used for a range of reasons with social interaction as one of the main reasons; however, it can be used for power, control, manipulation and management and each of these concepts are studies on their own. The issue of power is an important area as though paternalism (i.e. where the professional makes the decision for the patient) is said to have declined. Lupton (2003) argues that this is not the case and our approach could be described as tokenistic.

Almost any field in the domain of communication with its underlying theoretical underpinnings can bring a different understanding and different perspectives to the communication process.

A *critical social perspective* (Robb *et al.* 2004) considers issues of power, gender, inequalities and race as influential in the communication process. This understanding raises issues within the health care setting, for example do health care professionals engage in collaboration with service users or are there still power imbalances? If someone has English as their second language do professionals become impatient and shorten the consultation as it presents difficulties for them?

A *psychodynamic perspective* (Woolfe & Dryden 1997) would argue that the communication process can be influenced by the unconscious; in other words, past events may influence our perspective and understanding of any given event. If a service user had experienced in the past poor care within the health care setting and perceived the staff as hostile, a further admission would affect the communication covertly as the patient without realising may act defensively (as a way of protecting themselves) and the professional would respond accordingly without realising the negative effect this would have on the ensuing conversation.

When you examine a *behaviourist perspective* (Rungapadiachy 2001), it would be argued that as a result of experience behaviour changes and a positive and/ or negative reinforcer would increase/decrease the behaviour. This perspective is not so much interested in the why of the situation but how patterns of behaviour are learnt and maintained. If you smile at someone and he or she smiles back you are more likely to engage with that person on a regular basis than someone who ignores or frowns at you. It could be that learnt communication skills elicit a positive response and so are repeated and become the norm. This form of training is popular in many settings not just in the health care domain.

A *humanistic perspective* (Woolfe & Dryden 1997) or 'person-centred' approach emphasises the importance of the individual and his or her beliefs in self. The individual's values and beliefs can influence how the individual responds to a situation. Obviously this applies to service user and professional equally. Rogers's (1957) core conditions for effective interpersonal relationships will be discussed later in this chapter. The essence of a 'person-centred' approach can be found in the counselling domain and many of the key skills used in communication education have been applied to communication skills. Accepting a patient, for example, without judgement is one of the core conditions of a Rogerian perspective. This is not as easy as it sounds because the patient admitted for heart surgery has continued to smoke could easily provoke feelings of judgement and affect the communication process (Activity 1.3).

Key Communication Principles

Rogers (1957) provides some sound principles for effective communication that by accepting a person as unique and individual, accepting the individual without judgement and unconditional positive regard with empathy and with genuineness it can create a platform for rapport and effective communication. These principles, however, require closer examination if they are to be linked to clinical practice.

Each of us constructs our experiences in different ways and we store those memories in our minds and make sense of our reality by calling on those experiences. Each

---

Activity 1.3

Read again the four different perspectives and explore one of them in more depth specifically linking your findings to the communication process and record 2–4 key points that have increased your understanding of that perspective. Reflect on the impact of your findings and how it will influence your own communication skills.

of us will choose to filter an experience by acknowledging parts and ignoring other aspects of the incident. So two people could be in the same accident and one will remember one part of the story in a calm way and the other person will recount a much more dramatic picture and become very emotional. Rogers (1957) is highlighting the individuality of each person and the communication process needs to acknowledge that what you understand and what the service user understands may be completely different based on differing experiences and stored memories.

Accepting someone without judgement is a very difficult concept to consider. Each of us holds our own beliefs and values and if, for instance, fairness is a strong value and you believe everyone deserves the right to equal treatment, a patient who has received preferential treatment and/or has not been given the required care can affect the way you respond to the decision-maker. You may find yourself behaving in a slightly hostile manner, ignoring the person and/or making decisions about their code of ethics. Without realising it at some level the judgements we make can create barriers in the communication process.

Accepting someone with unconditional positive regard in a genuine way requires empathy and understanding. It is argued that only parents can claim unconditional positive regard for their children, and yet it is possible to accept a person without compromising your own beliefs and values by separating out the individual behaviour from the individual self. Unless you can own your own judgements it will be virtually impossible to be totally congruent in accepting another with empathy and unconditional positive regard. Some examples may be the patient who continues overeating whilst waiting for hip surgery; the patient who has been violent to his partner and is waiting to go into rehabilitation for a drug-related problem; the single mother who is on benefits and is failing to look after her young children.

Questioning is another key principle regarding communication. It is important to ask yourself as to what is the purpose of this conversation; if I hold this conversation what effect will this have on the other person. What do I need to say or do? Be clear of the focus and of the effects. So many communication failures could have been avoided if only some thought and planning had taken place prior to the conversation.

Questions can be leading (Burnard 1996) and full of assumption; we assume that we know what people are thinking, feeling and planning without even asking them. We ask questions that are value-laden, that is we make judgements: 'you don't do that do you?' Confrontation can be very useful as long as a sledgehammer approach is not used; however, going round the houses is not very useful either. Some areas of health care require a more confrontational approach; however, this can still be attained with respect for the service user.

Self-awareness

Understanding yourself and your response to situations can lead to improved communication skills. The barriers to effective communication are often generated by the individuals' own response to the situation in hand.

- *Feeling uncomfortable with the situation*: Sometimes we can find ourselves in situations that leave us feeling uneasy, and conversations may be shortened and/or ended so that we can make an escape. Providing that there is not a sense of danger, the reason for these feelings can generate from past experiences. If, for example, when you were a child you had an unpleasant experience whilst in hospital the situation you find yourself in may be acting as a trigger. Reflective practice can help in these situations by asking yourself the following questions: Is this more about me and my past experiences? Do I need clinical supervision to put things into perspective?

- *Personal issues*: If stress and anxiety are related to personal issues, our response to any given situation can be affected by the feelings and behaviours associated with stress. Being stressed can cause us to be irritated, curt and sarcastic, sullen and even voiceless if we cannot tolerate things any longer. Understandably, this will affect the communication process, and recognising our tolerance levels is important and developing strategies to manage stress levels is both important in the work place as well as in a more social context.

- *Feeling out of control*: When in a new situation you can easily find yourself feeling out of control; for example, you may have been asked to admit a patient and you have difficulty understanding the patient, and the more you ask for clarification the more you cannot understand. The feelings of being out of control will affect the interaction – you may need to cut short the procedure and seek someone else to continue or acknowledge to yourself that you are doing the best you can and complete as much of the process as is possible and report your difficulties to another colleague. As soon as you stop blaming yourself and recognise the situation as a challenge and that it is not about you being out of control, with all the accompanying negative self-beliefs this can generate, the sooner you will begin to feel more in control of the situation.

Self-awareness is the key to understanding the reason why some interactions are successful and why others are not. Realising how much our past experience can affect us and how certain triggers can generate a response that surprises us is a process that can take a long time. Concepts from the counselling domain can bring some understanding and this only reflects a simplistic macro overview, but it is worth considering when exploring the communication process. Issues of transference and counter-transference (Dryden 1989) bring understanding as to why some interactions fail.

Certain thoughts, feelings and actions can be transferred from patient to professional health carer; for example, maybe you remind the patient of a next-door neighbour who has caused them problems, and they treat you as if you are the neighbour, and this leaves you asking yourself why is this patient so hostile? Equally the counter-transference will be you behaving towards someone as if the patient is the individual in question. You will be aware of how often someone will say: 'She reminds me of my Nan/mother' and respond accordingly.

Another aspect of self-awareness is the boundaries we set on an interaction, and if there are issues of low self-esteem, a need to be liked, self-loathing, our conversations may be guided for a need to meet that concept of self. For example, you may be over-friendly in a professional setting and without those boundaries in place your need to be liked will be greater than your professional conversation.

Communication and Practice

When you first engage with a patient there are some core underlying principles that will enable this process. These same principles can be applied to relatives and other professionals. It is essential that you establish rapport and most of this will be achieved through the use of body language, facial expression, where you position yourself and touch. We are capable of picking up messages from body language – if someone is angry, depressed, grieving or happy, language is not required, and if you add facial expression the message is enhanced; yet, so many people are not aware of these messages. If you are in a strange town what makes you stop and ask someone for directions?

If you are approaching a patient, scan for those messages, and if the patient looks anxious, approach with empathy. Be aware of where you stand or sit, and if at all possible be at the same height as the patient as it can be very intimidating for the patient if you tower over them. Space is also an important consideration; often, we stand too close and may even touch the patient's arm as a means of comfort, but for some patients this action is intrusive, and this requires you to reflect on the question of touch and who is the touch for; is it to make 'us' feel better or is it for the patient's benefit? The question itself can make individuals defensive and state that of course it is for the patient. There are times when touch is appropriate but not all the time and not for all patients. When you observe facial and body language and act accordingly you will find that rapport will increase, as the message you give the patient is one of engagement. Watch how many times people carry on with other activities barely glancing at the receiver of their greeting and/ or information.

Always introduce yourself and explain all procedures, and when giving information ask the patients to explain what they think you have said, as it is often then that you discover that your explanation has not been understood. For some patients a conversation and a leaflet can help the process of understanding. For others, time and room for questions are required for comprehension. Yet others need the information in small chunks and others need time to think, find out more for themselves. If you accept the concept of being individual then it follows that information requires many approaches.

It is also important to listen to the tone of the voice, as it gives you many messages. When someone is sad you can hear the sadness in the voice, and equally if someone is happy this will also be conveyed through the tone of the voice. This can be important in telephone work as there are no visual clues. A patient can be telling you one thing, and the tone of the voice gives a different message. Equally, if you are able to recognise this, so can the patient, and if you feel irritated and/ or cross with the patient, they will be able to recognise this in the tone of your voice.

One of the most difficult aspects of good communication is the ability not only to listen but to hear. We can let people know that we are engaging in the conversation by the use of minimal prompts (Burnard 1996). We may nod our head or use para-language, for example 'mm'; however, the use of para-phrasing and summarising can let the person know that they have been heard, and it can also be an opportunity to clarify your own understanding. Following the told story, select the

Table 1.1   Closed and open-ended questions.

Closed questions (usually elicits a yes/no response)	Open-ended questions
Did you come on the bus?	How did you get here today?
Have you finished your treatment?	When will you be finishing your treatment?
Have you got any support at home?	What support do you have at home?

perceived key aspects and repeat it back to the person: 'So Mary you have been feeling unwell for 3 months and you say you are scared that there is something seriously wrong with you.' At this stage make sure you do not put any of your own interpretation as you may be completely right but also very wrong. Ask the individuals to express their feelings and accept their response; if Mary has told you she went to the doctors and she said it was nothing it would be easy to say, 'I bet you are angry with her' when this emotion has not entered Mary's head. This process of listening, hearing, feedback and asking more questions creates a forum for effective communication.

The use of open-ended questions can also generate a greater understanding of the issues being explored. As a principle, if you put who, what, when, where and how at the beginning of a sentence you will generate an open-ended question, and you can use 'why'; however, this can sound very judgemental and needs to be used with caution. The open-ended question, for example, can change the response you receive (see Table 1.1).

There are times when it is necessary to use closed questions, for example, when gathering personal details like name and address. With practice the use of open-ended questions will become a more natural way forward to improving communication skills.

Research: Communicating with Non-fluent-English-speaking Patients

Having presented some of the general theories of communication, the chapter now moves on to discuss some specific communication issues that have been reported. Gerrish (2001) reported that nurses found patients who could not speak English to be one of their greatest challenges. The United Kingdom is increasingly becoming a richer and more socially and culturally diverse society. Health professionals are therefore required to be conversant with the communication needs of patients who may not have been born in the United Kingdom and who may not have English as their first language. This does not mean that nurses need to speak multiple languages. What it does mean is that nurses need to be cognisant of the diversity of the population they serve.

Box 1.1 shows how a research study discovered issues relating to communication (Almond 2008).

> **BOX 1.1**
>
> **A study of equity issues within health visiting postnatal depression policy and practice (Almond 2008)**
>
> A qualitative case-study approach was used to study one PCT's health visiting postnatal depression service. Health visitors (HVs) were observed doing 21 home visits to antenatal and postnatal women. Post-observation interviews were conducted with 16 HVs. Nine Bengali women and 12 English women were interviewed. Additionally, 10 interviews were conducted with health visiting managers and other personnel involved in the health visiting postnatal depression service. In total, 51 interviews were conducted. The data were analysed using Ritchie and Spencer's (1994) Framework Analysis method.

The study found HVs had access to interpreters provided by a local authority. They could arrange to have an interpreter when they were visiting postnatal women in the home or when they saw them in the health clinic. The Primary Care Trust (PCT) had not placed any limits on how often HVs could use interpreters and indeed a local policy had clearly stated that the service needed to be equal and equitable. However, Almond (1998) found that HVs thought using interpreters was a costly resource. It took a lot of effort to arrange for an interpreter to accompany the HV on a home visit, and the visit itself was also more time consuming and challenging. Therefore, busy HVs were more inclined to use an adult member of the family as an interpreter. Yet, even when a professional interpreter was used, HVs lacked confidence in their ability to interpret accurately. The paradox is that resources were available but HVs were disinclined to use them. These findings echo those reported by Gerrish (2001), who reported inequalities in the care provided by district nurses to Asian patients. She too reported limited use of professional interpreters, and the disadvantages that Asian patients experienced because of poor communication between them and the nurse. She goes onto argue that district nurses need to acknowledge their responsibility to provide equitable services to all their patients irrespective of ethnicity and languages spoken. Equity can be defined as,

> Equity involves conscious and deliberate efforts to ensure and monitor whether appropriate services are provided and are accessible to those who stand to benefit the most from their uptake. This may involve making decisions that result in unequal distribution for some. Yet the standard and quality of services should be the same for all regardless of class, position race, disability, age, or gender. (Adapted from Almond 2002, p. 604)

Another barrier to effective communication was not related to the quality of the interpretation. The Bengali women said they did not want interpreters from the local community to be used. This was because they knew of instances where the interpreter had broken confidentiality and told other women about things she had been told at a home visit. So whilst the PCT had in essence attempted to overcome potential communication barriers, the actual resources provided were not culturally sensitive.

Activity 1.4

Read the case study below.

A case study of communication with a woman whose first language is not English.

Kishmiro is a young mother, who has been admitted to hospital for surgery. She arrived in England three years ago when she married her UK-born husband, Dharam. The nurse approached Kishmiro to carry out an assessment of her health. Whilst Kishmiro can speak English she does not speak it well. The nurse finds it very difficult to communicate with Kishmiro. She is not convinced that she has been able to carry out an accurate assessment. She tells Kishmiro that she would like her husband to interpret for her.

Read the following literature and then discuss the methods or resources the HV could use to communicate effectively.

Brooks N., Magee P., Bhatti G., Buckley E., Guthrie D., Moltesen B., Moore C., Murray A. (2000) Asian patients' perspectives on the communication facilities provided in a large inner city hospital. *Journal of Clinical Nursing* 9(5): 706–712.

Ledger S. (2002) Reflections on communicating with non-English-speaking patients. *British Journal of Nursing* 11(11): 773–780.

Meddings F., Haith-Cooper M. (2008) Culture and communication in ethically appropriate care. *Nursing Ethics* 15(1): 52–61.

Randhawa G., Owens A., Fitches R., Khan Z. (2003) Communication in the development of culturally competent palliative care services in the UK: a case study. *International Journal of Palliative Nursing* 9(1): 24–31.

Wells M. (2000) Beyond cultural competence: a model for individual and institutional development. *Journal of Community Nursing* 17(4): 189–199.

The HVs explained that they did not feel culturally competent and were therefore reluctant to do more than the minimum on visits to Bengali women. The immediate solution to these difficulties is HVs and indeed other nurses who lack cultural competence need training to give them the skills and knowledge to effectively communicate with their patients. Health professionals need translated literature so that patients can learn about their condition and treatment. It should not be assumed that people from low-income countries cannot read or write in their own language (Activity 1.4).

Robinson's (2002) review of studies involving interpreters concluded that trained interpreters can increase access to care but organisational barriers to their use need to be removed. The organisational barriers in Almond's (2008) study were the difficulties that HVs encountered in planning and organising visits with interpreters and the lack of an infrastructure to enable HVs to use interpreters from another city.

Ledger (2002) examined issues relating to bi-lingual student nurses and student midwives acting as interpreters in hospitals where they were receiving their training. She argues that this is an unsafe practice and can leave students vulnerable to being involved in discussions beyond their abilities. Nevertheless, the communication difficulties did lead to some innovative projects involving students and hospital staff developing multilingual and multicultural advocacy and communication resources. Randhawa *et al.* (2003) investigated the role of communication in providing culturally competent palliative care services in the United Kingdom. Their findings suggest that care is hindered by ineffective communication between health care staff and non-English service users. They also discuss the ethics and challenges of using family members as interpreters but found that link workers who were often used as interpreters lacked the skills to be involved in highly sensitive and emotional interactions between the staff and terminally ill patients.

Communication with Non-fluent-English-speaking Patients: Removing the Barriers

The application of communication theory here centres on communication with non-fluent-English-speaking patients. Theory without implementation remains no more than ethereal knowledge. Theory has to be used if it is to make a contribution to evidence-based practice and practice that is inclusive and culturally sensitive. As argued earlier communication is the main medium through which nurses and patients engage with one another. It is the means by which information is passed between both parties.

The following suggestions are provided as a starting point for communicating sensitively and effectively with patients who may not speak English or have limited ability in speaking and understanding English. They have been distilled principally from the authors' own experience of communicating with diverse communities and research involving participants who did have English as their first language (Box 1.2).

BOX 1.2

Overcoming language communication barriers in encounters with patients who do not have English as their primary language: 12 steps to more culturally competent practice

1. The patients' name can be an indicator that they may not speak English. When possible, contact previous health care givers to find out as much about the patients' spoken language, command of English, health beliefs and attitudes, dietary preferences and social circumstances. Find out which language they prefer to communicate in. Offer and gently encourage the use of a professional trained interpreter if the patients' or their own interpreter's English is not fluent. Check that you are pronouncing their name correctly.

2. When speaking keep the voice level moderate but speak slowly and clearly looking at the patient.

3. Keep sentences short and simple. Avoid using British idiom (for example, it's raining cats and dogs; I could eat a horse; my head's splitting). Avoid using nursing or medical jargon and technical language.

4. Be patient and allow time for the patients to form their sentence; remember that depending on the situation they or their interpreter will be translating what you are saying into their own language, then translating their response from their own language into English.

5. Use culturally sensitive and appropriate literature to communicate with patients.

6. Be guided by the patient's body language as to how formal or informal you need to be in addressing the patient. Take care with proximity, that is, the distance between you and the patient. This also includes eye contact and physical touch. A professional touching a patient's shoulder to show empathy, warmth and understanding is acceptable in most cultures. Do not assume if the patient is smiling or nodding that they fully understand what you have said. Ask for clarification.

(Continued)

BOX 1.2 Continued

7. Respect the patients' wish to have a relative with them during the nursing encounter.
8. Respect as far as possible the patients' privacy in respect to physical examination and sharing information.
9. Respect the patients' wish to be attended to by a male or female nurse.
10. Find out what the patients believe about their condition or illness as their beliefs may be contrary to the nurses own or professional beliefs. Explore sensitively and non-judgementally the patients' background, religion, dietary preferences and social arrangements.
11. Find out more about the culture of your patients and how best to nurse them by reading and talking to other health professionals who may have experience to share with you.
12. Use an interpreter who is not from the same community or town (in this country and their country of origin).

Conclusion

This chapter has explored the complex yet crucial essential skill of communication. By reviewing current health policy and the principles of communication skills, it has offered the reader a taste of this challenging area in terms of the client and patient groups you will encounter. The final section of the chapter captures some of the evidence base that is emerging on how nurses can play an active role in influencing communication and delivery of health care across a broad spectrum of people.

References

Acheson D. (1998) *Independent Inquiry into Inequalities in Health*. Department of Health, London.

Almond P. (2002) An analysis of the concept of equity and its application to health visiting. *Journal of Advanced Nursing* 37(6): 598–606.

Almond P. (2008) *A Study of Equity Issues Within Health Visiting Postnatal Depression Policy and Services*. PhD Thesis, Southampton University.

Almond P., Cowley S. (2008) Partnership: user involvement to improve health and wellbeing. In: *Public Health Skills: A Practical Guide for Nurses and Public Health Practitioners* (eds Coles L., Porter E.). Blackwell, Oxford.

Baggott R. (2000) *Public Health: Policy and Politics*. Macmillan, Basingstoke.

Brooks N., Magee P., Bhatti G., Buckley E., Guthrie D., Moltesen B., Moore C., Murray A. (2000) Asian patients' perspectives on the communication facilities provided in a large inner city hospital. *Journal of Clinical Nursing* 9(5): 706–712.

Burnard P. (1996) *Counselling Skills for Health Professionals*, 2nd edn. Chapman and Hall, Suffolk.

Department of Health (DH) (1998) *Saving Lives: Our Healthier Nation*. HMSO, London.

Department of Health (DH) (2000) *The NHS Plan*. HMSO, London.

Department of Health (DH) (2001) *The Essence of Care: Patient-focused Benchmarking for Healthcare Practitioners*. Crown, London.

Department of Health (DH) (2003) *NHS Modernisation Agency Report*. Department of Health. London.

Department of Health (DH) (2004a) *The NHS Plan: A Plan for Investment. A Plan for Reform*. HMSO, London.

Department of Health (DH) (2004b) *National Service Framework for Children, Young People and Maternity Services*. HMSO, London.

Dryden W. (ed.) (1989) *Key Issues for Counselling in Action*. SAGE, Bristol.

Equality Act (2006) HMSO, London.

Gerrish K. (2001) The nature and effect of communication difficulties arising from interactions between district nurses and South Asian patients and their carers. *Journal of Advanced Nursing* 33(5): 566–574.

Gerrish K., Husband C., Mackenzie J. (1996) *Nursing for a Multiethnic Society*. Open University Press, Buckingham.

Ham C. (2004) *Health Policy in Britain*, 5th edn. Macmillan, Basingstoke.

Ledger S. (2002) Reflections on communicating with non-English-speaking patients. *British Journal of Nursing* 11(11): 773–780.

Lupton D. (2003) *Medicine as Culture*, 2nd edn. SAGE, Bristol.

Meddings F., Haith-Cooper M. (2008) Culture and communication in ethically appropriate care. *Nursing Ethics* 15(1): 52–61.

Nursing and Midwifery Council (NMC) (2007a) *The Code: Standards of Conduct, Performance and Ethics for Nurses and Midwives* (implemented May 2008). NMC, London.

Nursing and Midwifery Council (NMC) (2007b) *Essential Skills Clusters*. NMC Circular 07(2007) Annexe 2, NMC, London.

Pincock S. (2004) Poor communication lies at the heart of NHS complaints, says ombudsman. *British Medical Journal* (3 January) 328:10.

Race Relations Amendment Act (2000) Office of Public Sector Information, available at http://www.opsi.gov.uk/acts/acts2000/ulpga_20000034_en_1 (accessed 12/11/08).

Randhawa G., Owens A., Fitches R., Khan Z. (2003) Communication in the development of culturally competent palliative care services in the UK: a case study. *International Journal of Palliative Nursing* 9(1): 24–31.

Ritchie J., Spencer L. (1994) Qualitative data analysis for applied policy research. In: *Analysing Qualitative Data* (eds Bryman A., Burgess R.G.). Routledge, London.

Robb M., Barrett S., Komaromy C., Rogers A. (2004) *Communication, Relationships and Care. A Reader*. Routledge, The Open University, Cornwall.

Robinson M. (2002) *Communication and Health in Multi-ethnic Society*. Policy, Bristol.

Rogers C.R. (1957) The necessary and sufficient conditions of therapeutic personality change. *Journal of Consulting Psychology* 21: 95–103 (reprinted in *Journal of Consulting and Clinical Psychology* (1992) 60(6): 827–832).

Rungapadiachy D.M. (2001) *Interpersonal Communication and Psychology for Health Care Professionals. Theory and Practice* (reprint). Butterworth Heinemann, Great Britain.

Townsend P., Davidson N. (1982) *Inequalities in Health: The Black Report*. Pelican, London.

Wells M. (2000) Beyond cultural competence: a model for individual and institutional development. *Journal of Community Nursing* 17(4): 189–199.

Whitehead M. (1988) *Inequalities in Health: The Health Divide*. Penguin, London.

Woolfe R., Dryden W. (eds) (1997) *Handbook of Counselling and Psychology* (reprint). SAGE, Melksham.

CHAPTER 2

Communicating with Children and Young People

Beth Sepion

Introduction

This chapter considers communicating with children and young people who are unwell and requiring a period of time in hospital. In order to communicate with children and young people, nurses require an understanding of childhood developmental stages and the potential impact of hospitalisation. This first section, therefore, begins with a review of the development of children's speech and associated ability to understand. Using this as a framework, communication strategies for the different stages will be explored.

The specific learning outcomes addressed in this chapter link with the Nursing and Midwifery Council's (NMC 2007) Essential Skills Clusters, and are identified below.

Learning outcomes

By the end of this chapter you will be able to do the following:

- Identify the key components of communication with children of different ages and stages of development.
- Define some of the qualities of effective communication with children and young people.
- Consider strategies to establish therapeutic conversations with children and young people.
- Consider factors that impact on communication with children and young people in the context of health care.

Communicating with Children and Young People

Nurses working with children and young people are required to establish trusting relationships in order to carryout day-to-day activities as well as unfamiliar and sometimes invasive, frightening procedures (Bricher 1999). It is essential, therefore, that they are able to communicate effectively with the child/young person however; as family-centred care is the basic ideology of children's nursing, they are also required to communicate effectively with adults. Corlett and Twycross (2005) identified that communication, and in particular negotiation, is still an aspect of practice that requires development in family-centred care. It is important to remember, therefore, that whilst the focus of this section is to explore the issues of communicating specifically with children and young people, it is always in the context of communication with the whole family (Coyne 2006).

Children and young peoples' ability to participate, and in particular to communicate preferences in health care, has been shown to have a positive affect on their care. However, they rely upon the support of not only the people around them, primarily their parents, but also health care professionals to be able to do this. Research specifically regarding communication with children in hospital is sparse, but there are two studies, Elliot and Watson (2000) which explored communication between health care professionals and children and Tates *et al.* (2002) which explored patterns of communication between general practitioners, parents and their children, which offer some guidance. Findings from Elliot and Watson (2000) identified significant issues for nurses, such as nurses listen more than doctors, they were perceived as being more approachable but less powerful. Other noteworthy findings were that they (children and young people) valued the opportunity to talk to someone in confidence about things that they felt unable to discuss with their parents and they wanted more information and confidential advice relevant to them. Tates *et al.*'s (2002) findings included views that parents generally considered their child's health as their responsibility and, therefore, did not expect the child to be involved in the consultation, and perhaps as a result of this only 5% of children were directly given information about their diagnosis and treatment.

Human Development and Communication

When considering a child's ability to communicate, it must be considered not only in relation to what would be expected for their age and level of development, but also in the context of the environment and circumstance, for example the stress of being in an unfamiliar environment, surrounded by strangers, perhaps in strange outfits can impact on children's ability to communicate or act as they would do at home. The symptoms of their illness will heighten their feelings and any parental anxiety may also be sensed by the child/young person and again this can influence their behaviour. Toddlers, preschool age and in particular school-age children are astute observers, picking up information when parents and/or health care professionals think they are engaged in something else. They read body language and compare facial expressions with tone of voice and the spoken word. Difficulties can occur if there is a mismatch between what they observe and what they hear. Children generally do not want to upset their parents and, therefore, they may feel unable to ask their parents questions that may cause them to become upset (Bluebond-Langner 1978). At home they may well have support networks – siblings, peers, significant others – that they can talk to, but in hospital they may feel alone and isolated, not knowing who to trust. A vital skill of nurses, therefore, is to read children's non-verbal cues, identifying changes in behaviour, recognising when there is a disparity between what they say or do not say and what their body language suggests.

Babies and infants (0–2 years)

Infants require exposure to human language and reinforcement in the form of adult positive responses at their achievement in order to develop language skills. Whilst in hospital it is paramount that this is maintained – nurses can encourage parents to continue to stimulate and interact with their sick infant. Communicating with this age involves being able to read non-verbal cues. The infants' posture, their facial expressions and body movements all give messages. Importantly, as they respond to adult non-verbal cues, when carrying out procedures or assisting with a procedure on an infant, it is important that they are reassured through the carers' body language – the tone and pitch of the voice, facial expressions and touch. Infants respond to higher pitch, but adults are recommended to use soft, gentle tones whilst maintaining eye contact without being intrusive.

Toddlers (2–3 years)

Between the ages of 2 and 3 years there is an acquisition of language, they know about 50 words, and it is the time that toddlers begin to assign meanings to words and start to construct two-word sentences. They are beginning to develop a sense of self and, therefore, want to have some feeling of control. Communicating with this age group requires patience, as the toddlers' thoughts may appear illogical; adults should encourage them to say the words that they know in order to convey what they mean. Offering choices helps them to develop their independence. As toddlers have a tendency to be possessive, communication may be more effective through admiration of a toy rather than a request to see their toy/book.

Pre-school age (3–5 years)

Pre-school children (ages 3–5 years) have the greatest acquisition of words. They can increase their vocabulary by up to 20 words a day. The important developmental aspect is their imagination. Their ability to misinterpret explanations and meanings of words make it paramount that adults ascertain children's understanding of words or procedures before they begin to explain new things. They are eager to learn things and often ask complex questions but equally have a short attention span so answers may need to be brief. In order to establish trusting relationships, it is vital that answers are truthful but with reassurance.

School-age children (5–10 years)

Children in this age group have begun to develop cognitively and are beginning to be able to use logical thinking. As previously mentioned they are astute observers

Activity 2.1

Read the following excerpt and then think about some other examples you may have seen or heard about. There may be friends or family members who have stories to tell that you may be able to associate with children and how they interpret adult communication patterns.

A 5-year-old thought he was dying because his parents were taking him to Disney. When he was first diagnosed he was in a bay with a 6-year-old patient who was going to Disney for her dying wish. They had talked about this and other things and 3 months later he, on being told of the trip as a treat for coping with the demands of treatment, concluded that he must be dying. He was unable to talk to his parents about this but when his unusual quietness prompted a nurse to ask if he was worrying about something, he was able to disclose his worry that he was dying.

and have a great need to make sense out of what is happening, especially when it is unfamiliar. Bluebond-Langer's seminal work in the 1970s identified that despite not being informed by parents or staff, children in hospital with cancer knew what was wrong with them and what was likely to happen to them (Bluebond-Langer 1978). They knew because they had observed their parents, the staff, other patients and they had talked to other patients – comparing signs and symptoms, treatments and outcomes. Bluebond-Langer identified the concept of mutual pretence where the children, for fear of upsetting their parents, did not ask questions and the parents interpreted this as them not wanting or needing to know. This study was with children with cancer, but it informs practice as to the importance of effective communication, as there is always the risk that children who are not informed may reach the wrong conclusion (Activity 2.1).

Adolescents (11–16 years)

This age group is often labelled as being 'difficult' or challenging to communicate with, and some staff feel unable or uncomfortable communicating with them, which can result in limited or stilted conversations leaving the young people believing that their feelings and opinions are not valued (Elliot & Watson 2000; Beresford & Sloper 2003). This was also identified by Sartain *et al.* (2000) in their study of 10–14 year olds with a chronic illness, who said that they were not listened to when they were in hospital. Further work by Forsner *et al.* (2005) discovered that the young people (11–18 year olds) described feeling hurt when health care professionals did not listen to them or treat them with respect.

Adolescence is a difficult time to be unwell. The impact on normal development is just as important as for the younger age groups, but the tasks of adolescence – developing independence, self esteem, body image – can create additional challenges for all involved. Whilst involvement in decision-making about their care is encouraged ultimately for those under the age of 16 years the legal rights remain with the parents or guardians (Rushforth 1999); this can result in poor compliance (Kyngas 2000). Therefore, effective communication with young people is essential if they are to be involved in the decision-making about their care and treatment. Kelsey and Abelson-Mitchell (2007) discuss how the type of language used can influence a conversation. In order for it to be a reciprocal discussion health care professionals have to use language that is understood by the young person. Earlier work by Catan *et al.* (1996) revealed that adolescents identified that being attentive, responsive, non-judgemental and a good listener as well as showing empathy were inherent skills of a good communicator.

Communication Strategies

Play is an important part of children's development, children learn through play; it represents normality. Therefore it is utilised in different ways. Mathison and Butterworth (2001) identified three different forms of play

- Normative
- Educative
- Therapeutic

Normative or everyday play in hospital enables the child to have a sense of familiarity and security.

Educative play is a way in which information can be given to a child. This can be in the form of books, comics and information DVDs (Weaver & Groves 2007).

Therapeutic play is used to help children gain an understanding of an event or procedure that is about to happen and also to gain insight into their understanding. The use of anatomically correct dolls, safe equipment enables the child to see, handle and experiment in order to learn. They may be encouraged to practice the event, taking a temperature on their teddy in order to appreciate what is involved (Weaver & Groves 2007). With younger children it is especially important for them to see, touch and feel things in order to make sense of these new experiences.

All of these forms of play, however, require effective communication to facilitate the child's participation. Building a trusting relationship with both the child and his or her parent is the first step.

Babies and infants (0–2 years)

Toys are useful in order to engage with babies initially and then to use as a form of distraction. However it is still essential, even though they will not understand what is being said, that babies are spoken to throughout procedures and interventions. As previously mentioned they will respond to facial expressions and the tone and pitch of the voice. It is important that they are reassured and comforted throughout interventions. The parents are the key people to do this, but it must be remembered that they may not be able to do this. In order for them to participate in such situations where distraction and immobilisation are required they need a full explanation of what is going to happen and how they can help, their role in the procedure can then be negotiated.

Toddlers (2–3 years)

Toddlers are developing a sense of self and, therefore, can demonstrate a strong will to be independent. Their ability to construct sentences requires patience as their mind often works more quickly than their mouth and they may appear to stutter. Engaging with this age group involves giving choices – 'which arm shall we use?' whilst avoiding closed questions such as 'Can I take your temperature'. Playing with the equipment, practicing on toys, parents or nurses enables them to gain trust and understanding. Encouraging their independence by asking them things such as 'do you want put the probe on your finger' also helps but patience is crucial as these take time while they master the skill (Weaver & Groves 2007). They are attuned to facial expressions and other non-verbal expressions, so it is necessary to monitor these whilst interacting with them. They are also good at listening when adults perceive them to be engrossed in other things, which mean that care must be taken not to discuss in front of them, things that could frighten or distress them. It is, however, vital, that everything that is going to happen to them is explained. This is where therapeutic play is invaluable. Finding out from the parent what they think their toddler knows already, what past experiences they have had and any coping strategies that they have previously successfully used will help to plan how the intervention can best be explained.

Pre-school age (3–5 years)

During this stage imagination and fantasy play an important part in development. This can lead to misinterpretation and misunderstanding of words for example dye and die. Clarifying their understanding of the words they are using is necessary. They can use the words in the correct context but not understand their meaning. For example they can use the word dead without understanding the concepts of death (Activity 2.2).

Play is the normal way for the pre-school children to learn, and the use of puppets, drawings and imaginative play helps them to show what they are thinking and feeling. Asking them to draw a picture of what happens in a hospital can be very enlightening (Herbert & Harper-Dorton 2002). This may be a way of getting to know a child and of engaging with them at a therapeutic level. Getting them to describe their pictures enables health carers to hear the words and terms that the child uses and may also facilitate an expression of feelings that this age group struggle with (Clathworthy *et al.* 1999; Wellings 2001). Honesty is crucial when explaining procedures/events to this age group.

Activity 2.2

How can you find out what pre-school children think and feel about the strange environment of the hospital? A member of your family or friends may have experienced this.

> **Activity 2.3**
>
> How might you find out what a school-age child understands about his or her admission to hospital? A member of your family or friends may have experienced this.

School-age children (5–10 years)

Whilst play is still important, school-age children will have begun to have experiences and therefore they may have an understanding of what is happening to them (Fosner *et al.* 2005). Tates *et al.*'s (2002) work identified however that health care professionals collect information from the parent rather than the patient (Activity 2.3).

With this age group particularly, it is important to find out what they think, know before explaining things. Questions such as 'can you tell me why you have come to the hospital today or can you tell me what is going to happen today'? provide insight into their understanding of what is going to happen and may also highlight misconceptions, for example, that they are ill because they did something wrong. It is not unusual for children to perceive hospitalisation or treatment as a punishment. It will also identify the words that they use which enables nurses to then use the same level of language.

This age group often respond to third-person conversations – using phrases such as 'other children have said that the mask smells funny'. This may enable them to talk about things that they feel they should be brave about. They are continually observing adult behaviour trying to make sense out of parts of conversations again with the potential of misinterpreting the conclusion.

Adolescents (11–16 years)

Deering and Cody (2002) suggest that adolescents perceive adults as being either caring and cool or insensitive and clueless. To establish a relationship with this age group, it is important to demonstrate respect for them. Key aspects of establishing a rapport with them is to listen carefully and to convey a non-judgemental attitude. This is done by using a neutral tone, phrasing and open body language, and by not responding to their sometimes 'shocking' or 'testing' tactics. However, Cooper (2006) suggests that two core skills to develop a therapeutic communication with adolescents and young people are free attention (Heron 1975) and active listening (Egan 1990).

Planning the interaction is important, expecting them to be willing and alert first thing in the morning if they have had a late night may not be a realistic expectation. Equally taking account of the environment – a four-bedded bay does not offer any privacy. Confidentiality is also important; however, it must be acknowledged that anything that is linked to their immediate safety will need to be explored further as to the reasons for needing to inform others, parents and the ways in which it can be done. Starting with questions about their peers or hobbies gives the nurse a chance to find out about the young person. Giving them a sense of control, asking them which they would like to do first, listening attentively, being comfortable with silences and using humour appropriately are valuable skills.

Kelsey and Abelson-Mitchell (2007) identified that in order to empower adolescents and young people in hospital health care staff need to talk to them using language that they understood. Non-verbal skills, body language, attentive listening was vital in order to establish a rapport and demonstrate respect for this age group. Good communicators were those who were kind and gentle demonstrating empathy (Fosner *et al.* 2007). They were willing to spend time with them, listening and answering questions.

Conclusion

Communicating with children and young people who are experiencing an episode of ill health requires special skills. It is important to remember that their ability to communicate may be affected by their illness, the environment and the impact of their illness on their parents. Their developmental stage must be assessed in order to utilise appropriate language and aids to establish a trusting relationship with them. To engage with toddlers, pre-school and school-age children, play can be a valuable and therapeutic intervention. For adolescents and young people, being willing to spend time with them, respecting their opinions and listening attentively to them are essential to gain their trust.

References

Beresford B.A., Sloper P. (2003) Chronically ill adolescents; experiences of communicating with a doctor: a qualitative study. *Journal of Adolescent Health* 33: 172–179.

Bluebond-Langner M. (1978) *The Private Worlds of Dying Children*. Princeton University Press, Princeton.

Bricher G. (1999) Paediatric nurses, children and the development of trust. *Journal of Clinical Nursing* 8(4): 451–458.

Catan L., Dennison C., Coleman J.C. (1996) *Getting Through: Effective Communication in the Teenage Years*. BT Forum, London.

Clathworthy S., Simon K., Tiedeman M. (1999) Child drawing hospital – an instrument designed to measure the emotional status of hospitalized school-aged children. *Journal of Pediatric Nursing* 14(1): 2–9.

Cooper M. (2006) Child and adolescent mental health. In: *A Textbook of Children's and Young People's Nursing* (eds Glasper E.A., Richardson J.). Churchill Livingstone, Elsevier, London.

Corlett J., Twycross A. (2005) Negotiation of parental roles within family-centred care: a review of the research. *Journal of Clinical Nursing* 15: 1308–1316.

Coyne I. (2006) Consultation with children in hospital: children, parents' and nurses' perspectives. *Journal of Clinical Nursing* 15: 61–71.

Deering C.G., Cody D.J. (2002) Communicating with children and adolescents: children are all foreigners. *American Journal of Nursing* 102(3): 34–41.

Egan G. (1990) The skilled helper: a systematic approach to effective helping. Brookes/Cole, California. Cited in Cooper M. (2006) Child and adolescent mental health. In: *A Textbook of Children's and Young People's Nursing* (eds Glasper E.A., Richardson J.). Churchill Livingstone, Elsevier, London.

Elliot E., Watson A. (2000) Children's voices in health care planning. In: *Evidence Based Child Health Care: Challenges for Practice* (eds Glasper E.A., Ireland L.). Macmillan, Basingstoke.

Forsner M., Jansson L., Soerlie V. (2005) The experience of being ill as narrated by hospitalised children aged 7–10 years with short term illness. *Journal of Child Health Care* 9(2): 152–165.

Heron J. (1975) Six-category intervention analysis. Human potential research project, University of Surrey/British Postgraduate Medical Federation, University of London, pp. 16–18. Cited in Cooper M. (2006) Child and adolescent mental health. In: *A Textbook of Children's and Young People's Nursing* (eds Glasper E.A., Richardson J.). Churchill Livingstone, Elsevier, London.

Herbert M., Harper-Dorton K.V. (2002) *Working with Children and Adolescents and their Families*. Blackwell, London.

Kelsey J., Ableson-Mitchell N. (2007) Adolescent communication: perceptions and beliefs. *Journal of Children and Young Peoples Nursing* 1(1): 42–49.

Kyngas H. (2000) Compliance of adolescence with chronic disease. *Journal of Clinical Nursing* 9(4): 549–556.

Mathison L., Butterworth D. (2001) The role of play in the hospitalisation of young children. *Neonatal, Paediatric and Child Health Nursing* 4(3): 23–26.

Nursing and Midwifery Council (NMC) (2007) *Essential Skills Clusters*. NMC Circular 07(2007) Annexe 2, NMC, London.

Rushforth H. (1999) Practitioners review. Communicating with hospitalised children; review and application of research pertaining to children's understanding of health and illness. *Journal of Psychology and Psychiatry* 40(5): 683–691.

Sartain S.A., Clarke C.L., Heyman R. (2000) Hearing the voices of children with chronic illness. *Journal of Advanced Nursing* 32(4): 913–921.

Tates K., Meeuwesen L., Elbers E., Bensing J. (2002) 'I've come for his throat': roles and identities in doctor–parent–child communication. *Child: Care, Health and Development* 28(1): 109–116.

Weaver K., Groves J. (2007) Fundamental aspects of play in hospital. In: *Fundamental Aspects of Children and Young People's Nursing Procedures* (eds Glasper A.E., Aylott M., Prudhoe G.). Quay Books, London.

Wellings T. (2001) Drawings by dying and bereaved children. *Paediatric Nursing* 13(4): 31–36.

Section 1

CHAPTER 3

Communicating with People with Learning Disability

Kevin Humphrys and Jane Smith

Introduction

This chapter briefly explores the nature and causation of learning disability and the impact this can have on effective communication through the exploration of growth, development, anatomical and environmental perspectives. From exploring these key determinants, application to practice is discussed with case examples provided and the skills of the nurse examined. This chapter also links with Chapters 1 and 6 and includes elements of care and compassion.

The specific learning outcomes addressed in this chapter link with the Nursing and Midwifery Council's (NMC 2007) Essential Skills Clusters, and are identified below.

Learning outcomes

By the end of this chapter you will be able to do the following:

- Briefly outline the nature and causation of learning disability.
- Consider key barriers to effective communication for people who have a learning disability.
- Describe different forms of communication and recognise the implications for effective interaction.

Effective Communication and Learning Disability

To be able to effectively communicate with other people is essential to our growth, health and social well-being. For those of us who are able to communicate effectively it is hard to imagine a world where our language, gestures and behaviour are continually misinterpreted or ignored by others. However difficult it is to imagine, this is a world that many people who have a learning disability find themselves in (Activity 3.1).

Activity 3.1

You are able to use the toilet, but on being admitted to hospital, you are fitted with a catheter without explanation. The catheter is not for medical reasons. How would you feel and how would you react? Take the same scenario but this time imagine you have no verbal communication and limited hand movement. Now how would you feel and react?

What is learning disability?

A learning disability is described as being

- a significantly reduced ability to understand new or complex information, to learn new skills (impaired intelligence), with;
- a reduced ability to cope independently (impaired social functioning);
- which started before adulthood, with a lasting effect on development.

(DH 2001, p. 14)

Mencap (2008, p. 6) states: 'A learning disability is caused by the way the brain develops. There are many different types of learning disability, and most develop before a baby is born, during birth or because of a serious illness in early childhood. A learning disability is lifelong and usually has a significant impact on that person's life'. A learning disability also has an impact on the way others view and interact with the person.

The attributed cause of the learning disability will be prior to the age of 16 and can be from biological factors, genetic or chromosomal; non-genetic causes such as infections or toxins and through environmental factors such as poverty or diet. It is estimated that there are 1.5 million people with learning disability in the United Kingdom (Mencap 2008). In 2001, the Department of Health (DH) calculated that 210 000 have a severe learning disability (DH 2001). It is reasonable to expect that this number has risen in the seven intervening years.

Whatever the cause, there is no cure. However, this does not mean that people should be treated differently from anyone else. What has to be considered carefully is the support the person needs from society, services and individuals, to enable them to live as independent a life as possible.

History to present day

History shows people with learning disability being stigmatised and segregated from main stream society. Through the late nineteenth and twentieth century many people with a learning disability lived away from home in large residential accommodations referred to as hospitals or institutions. During the 1970s, in the United Kingdom, these housed up to 65 000 people. This was typically a life of segregation and poor living conditions. Through the 1960s and until the late 1990s the living conditions and the general care that people received within these hospitals came into question. Inquiries into care practices at Ely Hospital (DHSS 1969), Farliegh Hospital (DHSS 1971) and Whittingham Hospital (DHSS 1972) began to be conducted. The move to close long-stay hospitals began with the

---

Activity 3.2

1. What behaviours do you think could indicate that someone is physically ill and in pain?
2. Now, think about this for someone who has a severe learning disability and no verbal communication?
3. What behavioural cues do you show if you are in a state of distress? What physical symptoms would you also notice?
4. How do these behaviours compare with those related to pain?

Mental Health Act 1959, followed by the government white paper, *Better Services for People with a Mental Handicap* (DH 1971) and the *Community Care Act* (DH 1990). Despite the move to close institutions and provide care in a community setting, services for people with a learning disability continue to underperform with stories of abuse and neglect now common within the media (CSCI and HCC 2006, HCC 2007a,b).

However, these inquiries are not just related to learning disability services. A recent report from Mencap (2007), entitled *Death by Indifference*, highlights the poor treatment received by six people with learning disabilities admitted to acute adult and mental health services. This poor treatment ultimately led to these peoples' deaths. The report goes as far to say that institutional discrimination exists within the National Health Service (NHS) towards people who have a learning disability with them getting worse health care than non-disabled people. One of the major concerns raised by Mencap was the notion of diagnostic overshadowing. This is neglecting to recognise signs and symptoms of ill health assuming them to be characteristic of a person's learning disability (Activity 3.2).

Death by Indifference (Mencap 2007) attributed the unacceptable standards of care largely to an ignorance or apathy by nurses and other health professionals to understand and listen to their clients with learning disabilities. It is important that the individual is continually consulted about their care regardless of the extent of their learning disability (DH 2005).

It is unrealistic to expect that in a peripatetic care situation health professionals would be able to understand every aspect of altered communication. What is important is that they recognise that someone is trying to communicate through an altered means. In trying to interpret someone's altered communication it may be that, in some cases, the person's carer and family need to be involved. Case study 3.1 demonstrates how a simple process, such as being weighed, for someone with limited experience of being weighed in a strange environment requires careful communication. Read this now before moving on to the section on Developing Good Communication.

Developing Good Communication

Being weighed can be seen as a simple process without the need for explanation. For someone with limited experience of being weighed in a strange environment, appropriate explanation was crucial. In order to facilitate an effective

---

Case study 3.1

An individual with a moderate learning disability who has a terminal illness is attending an outpatients clinic. This appointment is to monitor the client's condition and adjust care as necessary. The clinic nurse had to measure basic observations prior to the client being seen by the consultant. One of the observations was a recording of the person's current weight. The method of weighing the client was different to the client's expectations.

The client's immediate reaction was to scream and cry. The clinic nurse was shocked by the behaviour and tried to calm the situation by saying 'let's not bother'. The carer, experienced in interpreting the person's behaviour, explained to the clinic nurse that the person did not understand what was being asked and this was the client's way of communicating this. After an explanation to the clinic nurse, the process and reason was re-explained to the client in a manner that could be interpreted more effectively by the client.

Activity 3.3

What do you think the person with the learning disability was feeling at this time? Why do you think the clinic nurse reacted in the way she did? What could have been the care consequences if the clinic nurse's original reaction had been accepted?

---

communication process for people with a learning disability the nurse must have an awareness of their need to understand and interpret altered communication. This understanding may be the need to seek help from carers, family, friends and/ or interpreters. Furthermore, it is essential that we are non-judgemental towards a person or his or her behaviour. In Case study 3.1, the clinic nurse's behaviour was judgemental leading to avoidance by suggesting that the person is not weighed. By suggesting the person is not weighed, the clinic nurse hoped that the screaming and crying behaviour would stop. Such avoidance alters the nursing process. The incomplete assessment will lead to incomplete planning and subsequent inappropriate interventions.

This was clearly demonstrated in Mencap's (2007) report *Death by Indifference* (Activity 3.3).

The chapter has already explored that people with a learning disability are not listened to and are not given the information to make sense of what is happening. The result for the person with a learning disability can be that his or her needs go unmet, which can lead to fear, anxiety, resentment and withdrawal. For someone who has different communication abilities, these emotions can alter the communication further into something that is not recognisable by others. Behaviours can begin to escalate and it would be easy to read the communication as challenging behaviour and something to avoid rather than something to be listened to (Kevan 2003). By reading the communication as challenging there is a grave danger of ignoring the fact that it is highly probable that people who have learning disability are more likely to have other disabling conditions such as multiple complex medical problems coupled with their communication difficulties (Zwakhalen *et al.* 2004).

Activity 3.4

In this exercise we have provided some factors that impact on how a person may communicate. Spend time thinking about each of these and the impact it can have for all people within the communicative process.

- Phenotype behaviour (behaviours that are attributable to a specific syndrome or condition)
- A person's socialisation
- Nature and causation of the learning disability
- Sensory impairment
- Physical disability
- Perceived antisocial behaviour
- Involuntary behaviours (twitching, ticks)
- Verbal and reading ability, but little knowledge of concepts, that is on, over, 5 minutes.

It is already recognised that people who have a learning disability are more likely to have greater health care needs than those of the general population (DRC 2006, RCN 2006, HCC 2007b) and by labelling behaviour as challenging rather than communicative could in fact be ignoring someone's pain and discomfort. Communication is therefore more than just language; it involves signing, eye contact, facial expressions, gestures, body language and physical contact (Nind & Hewett 2001). Voice tonality is not considered as the main form of communication; it only contributes to 38% of our actual communication process and the spoken word only 7% with body language being 55% (Donnelly & Neville 2008). As a nurse we therefore need to be able to use our skills in innovative and creative ways to listen and give information in an accessible way that informs individuals and also elicits their views. Only when you do this are people truly participant in decisions relating to their own lives (Activity 3.4).

Altered Communication

For some people who have a learning disability verbal communication may be evident, but you may have to listen carefully to be able to fully understand what is being said. The clarity of the words may be compromised due to a physical disability related to the anatomical structure of the mouth and pallet. Here other professionals such as speech and language therapists may work with the person to help them develop their speech processes. On the other hand, the disability may mean that speech will not develop clearly and therefore a multimodal approach may be necessary to aid effective communication.

Verbal communication could be complemented with sign language, picture boards and computer technology. One sign language used by people with a learning disability is Makaton, which is based on British Sign Language but is more of an aid to communication rather than a language. Makaton uses speech and symbols to compliment the signs, hence providing the person with a range of options to support learning and the communication process. The important issue is that we are able to validate the communication to ensure that we do not get, 'the wrong end of the stick' (Porter *et al.* 2001). The authors explain that staff can assume they know the meaning that is being conveyed and under these circumstances it is important to keep checking that the inference of meaning is in fact correct. Porter *et al.* (2001) also refer to the fact that for some people, staff will be in continued disagreement as to the meaning of the behaviour as the nature of the communication methods can be idiosyncratic, that is behaviours and sounds have meaning that is specific to that person. For example, people with Rett Syndrome may place their hand in their mouth. This is a commonly displayed characteristic of this syndrome. Some staff, however, may associate this with hunger as it relates closely to the Makaton sign for hunger. Yet it could be that this is purely a phenotype behaviour (behaviours associated with the syndrome) or the person has tooth ache or some other health need.

Partners in communication and care

In generic health care services there may not always be the time to fully understand the person's idiosyncratic communication. Therefore, it may be necessary to involve family, friends and carers and possibly interpreters to begin to know and understand the person's communication. One key process in learning disability services that will help us in this is known as person-centred planning. Gates (2006) indicates that the central premise of person-centred planning is that individuals with learning disabilities are able to make choices about their lifestyle and once achieved, the role of services and professionals is to ascertain how these choices can be achieved. There is a danger, however, that person-centred planning becomes a tokenistic approach with people becoming recipients of well-meaning intentions rather than being participative themselves. There is also a risk of person-centred planning becoming a task-orientated exercise rather than an ongoing process of changing lives. The term person-centred means activities that are based upon what is important to the person from his or her own perspective and that contribute to his or her full inclusion within society (DH 2001).

To fully include a person it is imperative not to avoid situations we find difficult by finding something else to do that removes us from the cause of that difficulty (think back to the earlier case study of weighing the client). If you begin to attribute the difficulty to the person with a learning disability, then in fact you are compounding that person's disability by sending out a message to him or her that what he or she has to communicate and offer is not important. Read Tom's story in Case study 3.2 to gain a better understanding of all these issues.

Working with the person is therefore essential. This gives you time to observe and engage in what the person enjoys doing. This will also enable you to begin to interpret how their communication links to the activities, and by doing this you will be able to begin to associate the meaning of behaviours, signs and noises (Activity 3.5).

Nind and Hewett (2001) remind us that 'we are the resource that makes the communication partner' and further state, 'what takes place is going to take place because you use yourself well'.

Case study 3.2

Tom often lies on the floor and screams. This behaviour has not been assessed and the communicative function is undetermined. The staff response on this occasion is to ignore Tom because he always screams. However, Tom happens to be lying on the floor with a fractured femur because he has fallen down a step. A scream is not just a scream. There are different qualities, different volumes and different intonations. To not assess this is unacceptable because you are denying Tom the right to be heard, communicate and engage with others. The lying down may also have a communicative function, for example, feeling unwell, seizure, instability due to physical disability, hence ignoring the behaviour would be failing to meet his physical and psychological needs and a neglect to duty of care.

Activity 3.5

Now go back to the case study with the clinic nurse highlighted earlier in the chapter. Given the points discussed so far, how do you think the clinic nurse could have dealt with the situation better?

Conclusion

Many of the difficulties that people with a learning disability face when trying to communicate are related to external barriers. These include people's lack of knowledge of common language systems used, a lack of knowledge related to people's cognitive impairment, sensory impairment and physical impairments. Some staff and members of the society may well carry negative attitudes and have belief in myths such as eternal child, we know best, and the notion that people with a learning disability are violent. All of these factors will have a major impact on the development of a therapeutic relationship.

An understanding of the social context of behaviour, knowledge of social norms that govern expressive communication and a willingness to understand are crucial elements if effective communication is to be established. Personal interpretation of others' behavioural communication and perceived unconnected noises, such as grunts, groans and screams, can be functional communicative systems.

Those involved in the care of people with a learning disability must be able to support that person, ensuring person-centredness and real inclusion in the communication process. By doing this we can begin to identify a person's needs more effectively rather than basing needs on speculation, stereotypic notions and inaccurate information.

References

Commission for Social Care Inspection and Health Care Commission (2006) Investigation into the Service for People with Learning Disabilities at Cornwall Partnership NHS Trust.

DH (1971) *Better Services for People with a Mental Handicap*. HMSO, London.

DH (1990) *NHS and Community Care Act*. HMSO, London.

DH (2001) *Valuing People: New Strategy for Learning Disability for the 21st Century*. HMSO, London.

DH (2005) *Mental Capacity Act*. HMSO, London.

DH (2007) *Good Practice in Learning Disability Nursing*. Central Office of Information, London.

DHSS (1969) *Report of the Committee of Inquiry into Allegations of Ill-treatment of Patients and Other Irregularities at the Ely Hospital*, Cardiff Cmnd, 3975. HMSO, London.

DHSS (1972) *Report of the Committee of Inquiry into Whittingham Hospital*, Cmnd, 4861. HMSO, London.

DHSS (1971) *Report of the Farleigh Hospital Committee of Inquiry*, Cmnd, 4557. HMSO, London.

Disability Rights Commission (DRC) (2006) *Equal Treatment: Closing the Gap*. Background evidence for the DRC's formal investigation into health inequalities experienced by people with learning disabilities or mental health problems.

Donnelly E., Neville L. (2008) *Health and Social Care: Knowledge and Skills. Communication and Interpersonal Skills*. Reflect, Exeter.

Gates B. (2006) *Care Planning and Delivery in Intellectual Disability Nursing*. Blackwell, Oxford, UK.

Health Care Commission (2007a) Joint Investigation into the Provision of Services for People with Learning Disabilities provided by Sutton and Merton Primary Care Trust.

Health Care Commission (2007b) *A Life Like No Other*. A national audit of specialist inpatient healthcare services for people with learning difficulties in England.

Kevan F. (2003) Challenging behaviour and communication difficulties. *British Journal of Learning Disabilities* 31: 75–80.

Mencap (2007) *Death by Indifference, Following up the Treat One Right*! Report. Mencap, London.

Mencap (2008) *Mencap Manifesto: Making Rights a Reality*. Mencap, London.

Nind M., Hewett D. (2001) *A Practical Guide to Intensive Interaction*. British Institute of Learning Disabilities, Kidderminster, UK.

Nursing and Midwifery Council (NMC) (2007) *Essential Skills Clusters*. NMC Circular 07(2007) Annexe 2, NMC, London.

Porter J., Ouvry C., Morgan M., Downs C. (2001) Interpreting the communication of people with profound and multiple learning difficulties. *British Journal of Learning Disabilities* 29(1): 12–16.

RCN (Royal College of Nursing) (2006) *Meeting the Health Needs of People with Learning Disability: Guidance for Nursing Staff*. RCN Learning Disability Nursing Forum, RCN, London.

Zwakhalen S., Van Dongen K., Hamers J., Huijer H. (2004) Pain assessment in intellectually disabled people: non verbal indicators. *Journal of Advanced Nursing* 45(3): 236–245.

CHAPTER 4

Communicating with People with Mental Health Issues

Paula Libberton

Introduction

This chapter considers how to communicate with people when they are experiencing mental health problems. It is important to remember that everyone experiences mental health problems differently and that what is discussed here is a generalisation based on experience of working with people in this situation and from the literature which is available on this subject. The issues that will be explored include working with people who are showing depressive symptoms who may not be interested in communicating and may just want to die; communicating with people who are anxious to the state of panic and need you to take control; and exploring communication with people who are experiencing psychosis who appear to be in a different world. Any one of these groups of people may be difficult to engage because they do not want, are unable to accept or believe that they need help. As a result, this may lead to aggressive or threatening behaviour. This is acknowledged but not discussed in any detail in this chapter. Instead, what is advocated is the adoption of an appropriate philosophy of care which will ensure effective communication with anyone experiencing a mental health problem.

The specific learning outcomes addressed in this chapter link with the Nursing and Midwifery Council's (NMC 2007) Essential Skills Clusters, and are identified below.

> **Learning outcomes**
>
> By the end of this chapter you will be able to do the following:
>
> - Explore a philosophical approach which should underpin the care of someone experiencing a mental health problem.
> - Provide an overview of depression, the impact it may have on an individual and ways of communicating with someone experiencing these symptoms.
> - Discuss the concept of anxiety and suggest ways that it can be managed.
> - Identify the key features of psychosis and ways of supporting people through this often challenging experience.

Philosophy

In order to work effectively with people experiencing a mental health problem, it is important to be clear about the philosophy underpinning your approach to care. It is now well-recognised that people experiencing mental health problems are no different from the rest of the general population. Each person can be seen to be on a continuum with mental health at one end and mental ill health at the other end. Depending on what is happening in a person's life, in conjunction with their genetic composition and past experiences, that person can move up and down the mental health–mental ill health continuum (Greenberger & Padesky 1995). The person remains the same but their mental health fluctuates. Therefore, when caring for someone who is mentally unwell, it is extremely important not to loose sight of who they are when they are mentally well, and to keep this in mind when communication may appear difficult.

In addition to remembering that you or I could be that one in four people who experience a mental health problem each year (Office of National Statistics 2001a), it is necessary to consider what we believe the possible outcomes of this problem or illness to be. This belief will influence the way that we communicate with people. If you believe that everyone has the potential to recover from whatever problem or illness they are experiencing, you will have a chance of instilling hope in that person that there will be a successful outcome (Deegan 1992). This may not necessarily be cure, but it may be a move towards the place that the person would like to be, that is, emotionally, physically and spiritually. The demonstration of the hope that you have for this person's recovery is key to the relationship that you build in order to effectively communicate with that person during their period of ill health.

Communicating with the Depressed Person

People who are depressed often do not want to communicate. One of the contributing factors to a diagnosis of depression is a person's diminished ability to communicate, due to lack of interest or pleasure in activities they previously enjoyed and reduced levels of concentration, difficulty in thinking and making decisions (American Psychiatric Association (APA) 2000). Usually we talk about things that interest us and that we like doing. If your mood is so depressed that you no longer seem to enjoy anything then it may mean that you have little to talk about. This may be the main reason why someone who is depressed does not speak. Therefore, assisting someone in identifying a topic of conversation that does not require much thought may be a good starting point. This may involve talking about the current weather or what is going on outside. To the untrained eye it may seem that you are making meaningless conversation. However, if the person is having difficulty in concentrating and finding it difficult to think, there is little point in entering into a debate about his or her views on, for example, global warming. This is bound to put a stop to any communication that may have started.

Encouraging talking

Successfully engaging someone who is depressed in conversation is the first step to finding out what you can do to help. Often people who are depressed feel worthless (APA 2000). They do not think that they are worth talking to because they have nothing of interest to say. Therefore, it is important to show that you are interested in hearing their story before any judgement. This demonstration of curiosity about the person is often enough to start to increase a person's self-worth. Having someone interested in your story generally means that you are worthwhile. Asking open questions can assist the person in continuing their story (Greenberger & Padesky 1995) at the times when they may lose concentration or find it difficult to think. Examples of open questions include 'tell me more about that' and 'can you give me an idea of how you are feeling just now?' Sometimes the person may not answer your question, perhaps, because they did not understand it, or in the case of depression because they are not able. When people are very depressed, it is often difficult for them to say how they feel. However, their body language may give a good indication of the feeling that they are having difficulty in expressing. For example, someone who is finding it hard to make eye contact may be feeling ashamed about being depressed and needing help.

It is common for people who are depressed to talk negatively about themselves, their lives and their futures (Greenberger & Padesky 1995). It is often difficult to know how to respond to such negative statements without suggesting that they are incorrect in their views. Arguing with the person by saying that they are not worthless is unlikely to have the intended effect of making them feel more positive about themselves. Instead, it is useful to ask the person how they might respond to such negative statements made by their friend. The responses that are elicited in this way are usually beneficial in helping the person making the negative statements see another more positive side to their situation. Consider the statements in Activity 4.1 and possible responses.

Activity 4.1

How might you respond to your friend making these statements?
Nothing I do ever goes right.
Nobody likes me.
There's no point in me continuing – everyone would be better off without me.

BOX 4.1

Questions to ask to assess suicidal ideation. *Source*: WHO (2000)

1. Do you feel unhappy and helpless?
2. Do you feel desperate?
3. Do you feel unable to face each day?
4. Do you feel life is a burden?
5. Do you feel life is not worth living?
6. Do you feel like committing suicide?

If the person responds by saying 'pull yourself together!' try asking whether anyone has ever said that to them before and finding out whether it helped. Generally, this will not have been helpful, so you can then ask 'what else might you say to your friend?' This should result in a constructive dialogue with helpful responses which should increase the person's self-worth.

Suicidal thinking

People who are depressed often consider suicide (Williams *et al.* 2005). This is usually as a result of feeling hopeless about a situation as the present feels unmanageable and there seems no way out in the future. Therefore, the only option is death as this will end the pain of life. This highlights the importance of having an underlying philosophy of hope that everyone can and will recover whatever recovery means for them. It is essential that you acknowledge how someone is feeling however difficult it may feel to talk about someone wanting to end their own life. Talking about suicide does not make a person suicidal, and if you suspect that someone is suicidal it is vital that you ask. See Box 4.1 for questions to ask if you suspect someone is suicidal. People expect practitioners to be interested in their problems whatever they are, so it would be strange if someone who was feeling suicidal found that no one wanted to talk about it. Death by suicide continues to be a serious problem, with 1% of deaths in the United Kingdom in 2006 being the result of suicide (Office for National Statistics 2008). Therefore, any opportunity to prevent another death should be seized. Providing people with the chance to talk about how they are feeling may be sufficient to help them see another way out.

Communicating with the Anxious Person

Anxiety is a normal response to threat or danger; however, there are occasions when anxiety interferes with an individual's personal, occupational and social functioning to such an extent that it is disabling. The person may avoid certain situations, imagine that terrible things will happen or experience distressing physiological changes (Beck *et al.* 2005). About 10% of the population experience a level of anxiety which interferes with their daily lives with 2–4% having an anxiety disorder (Office of National Statistics 2001b). It is, therefore, likely that you will come into contact with someone who is experiencing a disabling level of anxiety. It may

> **Activity 4.2**
>
> Think about a time when you have been anxious. What was it like to be anxious? List the physical signs, your feelings and how you behaved. Note down what helped you feel better or what you would have liked someone to do to help you feel less anxious.

be that they are anxious about their medical condition or they have an underlying anxiety disorder which is worsened by the prospect of impending surgery.

It is useful to consider a time when you have felt anxious in order to have a better understanding of what you are aiming to achieve with someone who is in an anxious state. Look at Activity 4.2.

The key to communicating with someone who is anxious, whether this is mild, moderate or severe, is 'being with'. Often people who are experiencing anxiety feel out of control. Therefore, it is important that someone exhibiting a calm demeanour is there to take control of the situation. This person does not have to say anything but be there for when the person is ready to talk.

Anxiety and panic attacks

There are occasions when people become so anxious that they panic. They may feel so scared that they think that they are going to die. In fact, sometimes people think that they are having a heart attack when what they are actually experiencing is intense anxiety (Clark 1986). This state usually lasts between 5 and 20 minutes (APA 2000). In order to assist someone who is panicking, it is important to remove them from the cause of the anxiety if this is identifiable and possible. You should speak to the person in a firm yet reassuring manner letting him or her know that the anxiety will pass. Help the person to regain control of his or her breathing as hyperventilation will only make them feel more anxious as a result of the psychological effects on the body. Do this either by counting as the person breathes, for example, breathe in for two and breathe out for two, slowly increasing the gaps between breaths as the person calms down. Or encourage the person to breathe in and out slowly into a paper bag. Do not try to show them a new technique to manage their anxiety as it will only make them more anxious. Save this for a time when they are feeling calmer. Do not ignore them in the hope that their anxiety will subside naturally as this will only increase their distress and potentially the length of the anxiety attack.

Chronic exaggerated worry

There are people who experience chronic exaggerated worry that is more intense than the reality of the situation (Beck *et al.* 2005). People in this position value the opportunity to begin to ventilate their feelings and to talk about what is happening to them. It is useful to explore how the person has managed periods of anxiety before. It may be that the person wants someone in particular to be with him or her when he or she is in this state. If it is possible then you could arrange for that person to visit or for him or her to go to see that person. They may manage by writing down their thoughts and feelings in a book that they can choose to close to reflect

---

Activity 4.3

Additional reading and resources

Bourne E., Brownstein A., Garano L. (2004) *Natural Relief from Anxiety: Complimentary Strategies for Easing Fear, Panic and Worry*. New Harbinger Publications, California.

This book outlines a number of methods for managing anxiety that do not involve prescribed medication. It includes relaxation techniques such as progressive muscle relaxation.

Harrison A., Hart C. (2006) *Mental Health Care for Nurses: Applying Mental Health Skills in the General Hospital*. Blackwell, Oxford.

This book is targeted at non-mental health staff. It aims to enable an understanding of patients' psychological and mental health needs.

---

on later when they are feeling less anxious. Or they may benefit from progressive muscle relaxation, which involves tensing and relaxing muscles systematically throughout the body to achieve a state of relaxation (Jacobson 1974). See Activity 4.3 for examples of relaxation techniques. There are many ways of communicating with someone when they are anxious but the key is to be there for them and to engage in activities that have helped in the past. If you follow these simple steps you will find that communication is easy and effective.

Communicating with the Psychotic Person

Communicating with someone experiencing symptoms of psychosis may be considered difficult and challenging purely because psychosis is a condition that most people feel far removed from. The reality is that all of us have heard voices (Kingdon & Turkington 2005) – do you remember when you were drifting off to sleep and you thought you heard someone talking downstairs only to find no one was there. How about the day you forgot to clean your teeth and you were paranoid that everyone was looking at you thinking 'how disgusting' when actually no one knew you had not cleaned them. Hearing voices and paranoid delusions are both symptoms of psychosis (APA 2000) which may suggest that the person is experiencing a different reality to the one that we know. Imagine how distressing it would be to have voices in your head condemning your every move or feeling so paranoid that someone was out to kill you that you feared for your life. It is this distress that makes people with psychosis behave in unexpected and sometimes difficult to explain ways.

According to Rogers (1983), empathic understanding, genuineness and unconditional positive regard are the guiding principles that underpin any successful therapeutic relationship. It is essential that these principles are followed to allow effective communication to take place. People need to feel safe to disclose significant and often distressing information (Romme & Escher 2000) and need to know that their experiences and needs will be taken seriously (Sainsbury Centre 1998). This is particularly important when what is being experienced appears different from the norm, as is the case in psychosis.

In order to display empathic understanding, it is essential to take time to listen to what the person is saying. This involves concentrating on what is being said, summarising what is said without changing the meaning and considering the content within the context that it is presented (Egan 2007). It may seem difficult to dedicate time to someone who appears to be making little sense (e.g. they are responding to voices so you cannot follow their conversation), when there are many other matters which require attention. However, this time and attention will allow you to develop a much better understanding of the person's needs and strengths, which is vital to any intervention that may be required. This attention will form the basis of any future effective communication.

Seating arrangements

When listening and talking to someone who is experiencing psychosis, it is particularly important to think about your seating arrangements. Sitting behind a desk is often seen as threatening with the person behind the desk appearing to be in a position of power and control (Dickson *et al.* 1997). In order to demonstrate empathic understanding it would be more appropriate to remove any barriers. Sitting on similar chairs suggests that both people are equal and placing the chairs at a 60° angle allows for easy eye contact, which is akin to most normal social interactions (Argyle 1975). Eye contact is essential for good communication. Poor eye contact suggests that something is wrong with long periods (over 70%) of intense eye contact often interpreted as confrontational (Barker 2003). If someone is feeling paranoid, gazing at them for prolonged periods may be construed as threatening and may provoke an aggressive response. It is therefore sensible to try and position yourself so that your exit is clear to leave the room if an undesired reaction is inadvertently provoked (Woodward *et al.* 2004).

Psychosis and aggression

Very few people experiencing psychosis are aggressive without provocation. Usually aggression is the result of one person trying to get the other to comply with something that he or she does not deem appropriate at that time (NICE 2005). Therefore, we need to put ourselves in that person's shoes and consider the ways that we might react to a given interaction. Activity 4.4 will help you explore this further. This should make us think about the potential effect our method of communication will have on that person. Sometimes the way we view people can have an effect on the way we treat them. It is therefore essential that we remember the principle of unconditional positive regard, which Rogers (1983) defines as accepting that all individuals are entitled to respect and care. At a time when we cannot understand why someone is behaving in a particular way, it can be easy to forget this important principle. We need to remain open and hopeful that the person will recover. This requires genuineness on our side that the person knows himself or herself best, his or her choices are of paramount importance and he or she has many strengths to go with the problems that he or she is currently experiencing (Gamble 2006).

Activity 4.4

1. Think of a time when you were feeling distressed, vulnerable or out of control.
2. List five different ways that people may have communicated with you at that time.
3. Note down how you may have reacted to those five different approaches.
4. Reflect on these approaches and possible reactions.
5. Consider how this might influence your future communication with someone who is mentally unwell.

BOX 4.2

Managing unusual beliefs

Service user: 'I am frightened of the rat in my stomach'.

Response which acknowledges how the person feels.
Practitioner: 'It sounds like you are feeling very scared of what is happening'.

Response which would reinforce the delusion.
Practitioner: 'It sounds like the rat in your stomach is very frightening'.

Response which would be seen as argumentative and jeopardise the therapeutic relationship.
Practitioner: 'Don't you realise a rat in your stomach would suffocate?'

Service user: 'Do you believe me when I say there is a rat in my stomach?'

Response which neither reinforces nor confronts the delusion.
Practitioner: 'I cannot see or feel the rat in your stomach, but I believe it is real to you'.

Unusual beliefs and hearing voices

People who are unfamiliar with working with individuals who are hearing voices or who have unusual beliefs often want to know how to react in these situations. The key is to remember the guiding principles of any therapeutic relationship: empathic understanding, genuineness and unconditional positive regard (Rogers 1983). These principles will ensure that you listen effectively to the person's distress with curiosity about how they are feeling. If someone is talking about a voice which you cannot hear, do not argue with them suggesting that they are mistaken; instead, focus on the feeling that it has evoked in them (Romme & Escher 2000). This feeling is very real even if the voice is not. The same premise applies to communicating with people who have delusional beliefs. Agreeing with the person's delusion is unhelpful while disagreeing will only serve to frustrate the person and increase his or her distress (Nelson 2005). Instead, focus on what appears true to you. See Box 4.2 for examples of ways of communicating with someone experiencing a delusion.

Conclusion

Communicating with people who are experiencing mental health problems can be challenging. However, adopting the right philosophy is key to providing effective support. Remembering that people with mental health problems are like you and I, and should be treated the same way that we would want to be treated is vital. At the same time we need to remember that people are individuals with their own needs. Suggestions can be made about communicating with people with specific mental health problems but ultimately it is our ability to provide empathic understanding, genuineness and unconditional positive regard along with curiosity and hope that makes for a successful and fulfilling outcome for both parties involved.

References

American Psychiatric Association (APA) (2000) *Diagnostic and Statistical Manual of Mental Disorders*, 4th edn. Text revision. (DSM-IV-TR) American Psychiatric Association, Washington.

Argyle M. (1975) *Bodily Communication*. Methuen, London.

Barker P. (2003) Interviewing as craft. In: *Psychiatric and Mental Health Nursing: The Craft of Caring* (ed. Barker P.). Arnold, London.

Beck A., Emery G., Greenberg R. (2005) *Anxiety Disorders and Phobias: A Cognitive Perspective*. Basic Books, New York.

Clark D. (1986) A cognitive approach to panic. *Behaviour Research and Therapy* 24: 461–470.

Deegan P. (1992) The independent living movement and people with psychiatric disabilities: taking back the control of our own lives. *Psycho-social Rehabilitation Journal* 15: 3–19.

Dickson D., Hargie O., Morrow N. (1997) *Communication Skills Training for Health Professionals*. Chapman and Hall, London.

Egan G. (2007) *The Skilled Helper: A Problem-management and Opportunity-development Approach to Helping*. Thomas Brooks/Cole, Belmont.

Gamble C. (2006) Building relationships: lessons to be learnt. In: *Working with Serious Mental Illness: A Manual for Clinical Practice* (eds Gamble C., Brennan G.). Elsevier, London.

Greenberger D., Padesky C. (1995) *Mind Over Mood: A Cognitive Treatment Manual for Clients*. Guildford Press, New York.

Jacobson E. (1974) *Progressive Relaxation*. University of Chicago Press, Chicago.

Kingdon D., Turkington D. (2005) *Cognitive Therapy of Schizophrenia*. Guildford Press, New York.

Nelson H. (2005) *Cognitive-behavioural Therapy with Delusions and Hallucinations: A Practice Manual*. Nelson Thornes, Cheltenham.

NICE (2005) *Violence: The Short-term Management of Disturbed/violent Behaviour in In-patient Psychiatric Settings and Emergency Departments*. NICE, London.

Nursing and Midwifery Council (NMC) (2007) *Essential Skills Clusters*. NMC Circular 07(2007) Annexe 2, NMC, London.

Office for National Statistics (2008) *Suicide Rates in the UK 1991–2006*. General Register Office for Scotland, Northern Ireland Statistics and Research Agency, available at http://www.statistics.gov.uk/cci/nugget.asp?id=1092 (published online 25/01/08).

Office of National Statistics (2001a) *Mental Health among Adults*. National Statistics, London, available at http://www.statistics.gov.uk/pdfdir/mhaa1201.pdf (accessed 09/04/08).

Office of National Statistics (2001b) *Psychiatric Morbidity among Adults Living in Private Households*. HMSO, London, available at http://www.statistics.gov.uk/downloads/theme_health/psychmorb.pdf (accessed 11/04/08).

Rogers C. (1983) *Freedom to Learn for the 80s*. Merrill, USA.

Romme M., Escher S. (2000) *Making Sense of Voices: A Guide for Mental Health Professionals Working with Voice Hearers*. Mind Publications, London.

Sainsbury Centre (1998) *Keys to Engagement*. Sainsbury Centre for Mental Health, London.

Williams J., Crane C., Barnhofer T., Duggan D. (2005) Psychology and suicidal behaviour: elaborating the entrapment model. In: *Prevention and Treatment of Suicidal Behaviour: From Science to Practice* (ed. Hawton K.). Oxford University Press, Oxford.

Woodward N., Williams L., Melia P. (2004) Creating and maintaining a safe environment. In: *Mental Health Nursing: Competencies for Practice* (eds Kirby S., Hart D., Mitchell G.). Palgrave Macmillan, Basingstoke.

World Health Organisation (WHO) (2000) *Preventing Suicide: A Resource for General Physicians*. WHO, Geneva.

CHAPTER 5

Communication and Loss

Carmel Sheppard and Pauline Turner

Introduction

This chapter considers some of the key communication issues in working with individuals and families who are affected by serious illness and other life-changing events. It will cover key principles that can be applied to the different settings in which people are cared for. Although much of what has been written about communicating in serious illness and at the end of life is based within the field of cancer and palliative care, a high proportion of patients in critical care settings will not recover and so effective and sensitive communication is a key requirement for health care professionals working in these areas. There may be different challenges for these practitioners, however, compared to those working in a hospice or caring for people at home or in a nursing home, and we will explore what some of these might be. Later in the chapter we will look at some of the guiding principles for practice in relation to working with people facing loss, communicating with children and other vulnerable people, responding to anger and denial and talking about 'bad news'.

The specific learning outcomes addressed in this chapter link with the Nursing and Midwifery Council's (NMC 2007) Essential Skills Clusters, and are identified below.

Learning outcomes

By the end of this chapter you will be able to do the following:

- Identify the key components of communication in advanced and life-threatening illness.
- Define some of the qualities of compassionate communication.
- Consider how people may be supported through adjustment to loss.
- Consider specific communication challenges including responses to anger and denial, talking about bad news and talking to children. See Activity 5.1.

> **Activity 5.1**
>
> At the start of this chapter take a moment to think about where seriously ill and dying patients might be cared for and what some of the communication challenges might be in the different settings. Then look at some of the key ones outlined in Boxes 5.1 and 5.2.

> **BOX 5.1**
>
> **Communication challenges in the acute and critical setting**
>
> One of the central conflicts in the critical and acute setting might be about the tension between the need to intervene and treat versus knowing when it is appropriate to allow someone to die. Some of the challenges here may be about explaining the benefits or otherwise of treatments and interventions and engaging in decision-making with close relatives and the medical team about end of life decisions. Another challenge might be the demands on time required by patients who are going to get better versus spending time listening and talking to those for whom 'nothing more can be done'. There may be difficulties in knowing how to communicate with unconscious or sedated patients. Shift-working patterns may also interrupt the continuity of communication with very ill patients.

> **BOX 5.2**
>
> **Communication challenges in caring for people in hospices or at home**
>
> The environment here may be much more conducive to spending time with people and listening to their individual preferences and concerns. However, some of the challenges may include how we might respond to awkward questions and ongoing information needs in relation to bad news. It is normal to feel at a loss for words when someone asks if they are going to get better after a poor prognosis has been indicated, and yet this often will be very uncomfortable for the professional. We may also be faced with patients and families who are angry and hostile or who may have a lot of emotion to vent.

Caring for People Who Cannot Speak

Nurses and health care professionals will care for people experiencing many different sorts of losses. More specifically to this chapter, they will care for people who have lost the ability to communicate in usual ways – for example, they may have had a tracheotomy or laryngectomy or may be ventilated or sedated; they may be aphasic as a result of stroke; they may be unable to speak audibly because of frailty or weakness; they may not be easily understood because they have a condition like dementia or a severe learning difficulty; they may not speak the same language. Happ (2000) calls this 'voicelessness' – the inability to communicate thoughts, feelings, desires and needs fully to others – and describes the impact this has on the process of care. It causes fear and anxiety, and a sense of powerlessness and isolation in patients; it profoundly affects the relationship which the family has with the patient at a crucial time; it makes the decision-making and care-giving process much harder for health care professionals (Happ 2000).

> **Case study 5.1**
>
> Joe, aged 58, had a brain tumour which had affected his speech. A nurse who was assessing his needs reflected on her discomfort at continually asking him to repeat what he was saying, and he also appeared to be agitated by this. His wife was with him and the nurse decided to ask if he would mind if she 'interpreted' for him. His evident relief demonstrated that he was happy with this request and his wife confirmed that she was close to him and had developed an ability to understand him very well.
>
> This might not always be the case and it is important to check that someone is happy to allow someone else to speak on his or her behalf. Another strategy that this nurse might have employed would have been to have used an agreed 'yes' and 'no' indication system (Hemsley *et al.* 2001).

Happ's study is essential reading for practitioners because it raises key issues for nurses working in many different types of setting with patients who are unable to communicate verbally and suggests that nurses have a key role in mitigating the detrimental effects of voicelessness. This may involve quite complex communication skills such as acting as an advocate or interpreter not only for the patient and family but also between the patients and their families when priorities differ; developing non-verbal communication strategies and supporting family members who may speak on behalf of their close relative but who are not prepared for this complex and emotionally taxing role (Happ 2000). Working with seriously ill people requires confidence in communicating (acquired through developing good skills in this area) and will inevitably draw upon practitioners' personal qualities and their values of care (Case study 5.1).

Compassionate Communication

Most of us would recognise the value of compassionate communication as opposed to communication which is mediated by someone who is distracted or disengaged from the meaning and impact of what is being said. Communication has with it a therapeutic component – it can make people feel better. Conversely, it can leave them feeling much worse. Levy (2001) describes meaningful communication as the process by which the dignity of patients and their families can be reawakened or rekindled. Thorne *et al.* (2005a) underline the fact that what is important to people is being known as a unique individual. This is of vital importance in a modern health care system in which health care professionals have many competing demands on their time and patients may feel depersonalised as a result.

Compassionate communication is focused on the patient and does not necessarily involve a lot of time. A patient commented: 'She [the doctor] was extremely busy, but the three minutes she had with you she was totally focused on you … and it was never the medical stuff, it was "how are you feeling?" ' (Thorne *et al.* 2005a). It is the value that we give to another person by listening to them and acknowledging that their experience is unique to them that makes communication so effective when people are facing loss. It inevitably involves a degree of relationship and connection with that person and has to do with our attitudes to people. 'A person is a person because of people' writes Heyse-Moore (1996, p. 305). In other words, it is the value and respect that we give to each other that enhances or diminishes us as people and this is reflected in the way we communicate. 'You matter because you are you' was a phrase used by Cicely Saunders who was one of the pioneering founders of the modern hospice movement to capture the importance of individualised care and attention (Saunders 1965).

Thus, the strength of the nurse–patient relationship is not necessarily just to do with the practical aspects of care but the overall therapeutic relationship inclusive of psychological care and the ability to form an intimate relationship based on trust, mutual respect and honesty. In difficult circumstances, this relationship together with the act of support and just 'being there' is the greatest contribution to care that we can offer to the patient.

In a study examining patients' experiences of communication with physicians, behaviours ranked as important to patients included communication based on active listening, awareness of the patient's depth of knowledge about their illness, honesty, the feeling of partnership, an overt interest in the patient as a person and an attitude of curiosity about the patient's needs, saying something realistically hopeful, validating concerns and eye contact (Harris & Templeton 2001). The use of touch was also considered important in this paper; however, it is important to recognise that this may be different within some cultures and that some patients may feel an invasion of personal space. The nurse who rushes to hold the patient's hand or demonstratively comfort the patient could be conveying a feeling of desperation which may result in increased anxiety for the patient. However, there is clear indication that touch tends to signify human connection within the health care relationship and is welcomed (Thorne *et al.* 2005a) (see Activity 5.2).

Avoiding Communication

The district nurse who was honest enough to express her feelings when she said: 'I find it awkward talking to patients who are dying. I don't know how to respond to some of the things they say like 'I haven't got long left' or 'Am I dying?' (Dunne *et al.* 2005) is unlikely to be alone in her discomfort. Existential questions of this nature are understandably challenging for most, if not all, professionals. Doctors and nurses are trained in different ways to 'make people better' and we

---

Activity 5.2

Read Gerald Humphreys's story about having lung cancer in Humphreys (2000). In this articulate account he relays the powerful feelings he had during his cancer journey that, however, seemed outside the awareness of the highly trained clinicians who were involved in his treatment. This article is followed by a response from a medical oncologist who did not participate in his care but who presents a perspective from the health care team's point of view. Reading patient accounts can help us to develop more awareness about how we communicate and what is important to people.

> **Case study 5.2**
>
> A man who had been told he had a 'tumour of the lung' discussed his illness with a community palliative care nurse. Although the doctor had said it was a 'malignant tumour' the patient had not immediately related this to cancer. As time went on, however, he had begun to wonder if it was cancer, partly because of the way health care professionals related to him – 'the "look" said it all'. The nurse asked him what he understood by cancer and he replied that it was something that 'ate away' at the whole body, rather than being confined to one place. The way he had understood a 'tumour' was that it was located in one place. 'Cancer', on the contrary, held much more terrifying images for him.

feel uncomfortable when people do not get better. Levy (2001) suggests that the ability to deal with uncertainty comprises much of the work with ill and dying people and yet health care professionals do not receive training in this.

It is not surprising, then, that there is substantial evidence from the literature that when faced with situations that require difficult communication some health care professionals use blocking or avoidance behaviours, such as the use of closed questions and the avoidance of difficult subjects which may elicit emotional reactions. (Wilkinson 1991; Maguire 1999; Hack *et al.* 2005; Thorne *et al.* 2005b). Some doctors may use euphemisms such as 'spots on the liver', 'lesion', 'growth' and so on which may be confusing for the patient (Chapman *et al.* 2003). In a review of the literature about communication needs and goals of cancer patients (Hack *et al.* 2005), there was found to be a wide variability in the degree of patient understanding particularly in relation to the extent and spread of their disease and the purpose of treatment. Even when patients have been given facts about their illness they may not have understood certain implications or they may hold misconceptions from other sources as Case study 5.2 illustrates. Having more than one opportunity to talk things through with professionals is thus very important.

There are universal difficulties inherent in communicating with ill and dying people – it is not just restricted to the cancer and palliative care field. De Araujo and da Silva (2004) cite similar barriers in their study based in a Brazilian intensive care unit. Although the nurses in this study recognised the importance of communicating with dying patients, they described an inability to 'know what to say' to patients who are sedated. This is supported in studies conducted in several countries (Green 1996; Happ 2000; Alasad & Ahmad 2005). And yet it is widely known that it is impossible not to communicate when you are caring for someone who is ill – it will happen through non-verbal messages, body postures, gestures, glances, absence or presence, tone of voice and touch (de Araujo & da Silva 2004). Compassionate communication is all the more needed when words are less dominant – critical care nurses need to employ patience, persistence and creativity in overcoming communication barriers (Happ 2000).

It is important to remember that effective communication is reciprocal – it is not just the responsibility of the professional. Clearly, the patient has a part to play in this, and Jarrett and Payne's work (Jarrett & Payne 1995) looked at ways in which patients also may resist talking to professionals about certain topics.

Activity 5.3

Further reading

For a discussion on communication skills within the palliative care setting and a focus on being partners in care with patients see Jarrett N., Maslin-Prothero S. (2004) Communication, the patient and the palliative care team. In: *Palliative Care Nursing. Principles and Evidence for Practice* (eds Payne *et al.*). Open University Press, Maidenhead, UK, 142–162.

Also read Mary Happ's participant observation study of critically ill, ventilated patients which describes the effects that not being able to speak have on families and professionals as well as the patients themselves (Happ 2000).

Other patients may not have the language or the skills to express how they are feeling and may need help in identifying their concerns (Activity 5.3).

Talking and Listening to Individuals and Families Facing Loss

People who are facing loss are usually part of a wider social network which involves family and friends. Our communication must always reflect this and from the outset we should consider, together with the person who is affected, who will need to be included in information sharing and what might need to be covered. Many patients fear the impact that their illness will have on their families more than the impact on themselves, and it is true that the intensity of being alongside a seriously ill relative can take its toll. Becker (2001, p. 186) cites an old saying: 'It is the patient who experiences the symptoms while it is the family who experience the illness' and care for the family is as important a consideration as for the patient. Offering a support system to help the family cope and using a team approach to address the needs of patients and their families is one of the stated aims of palliative care (Sepulveda *et al.* 2002) and will require an understanding of how loss and change may affect them and consequently our communication with them.

People experience loss in many different ways. The old English word 'bereafian' (from which we get our word bereavement) means to be 'robbed', 'dispossessed', 'left desolate' (*Concise Oxford Dictionary*, 8th edn, 1991). People may be left with a feeling of having been 'robbed' through losses, other than death. For example, a person may have suffered an injury (whether physical or psychological) that may leave him or her feeling robbed of a part of themselves. Or they may have lost their home, their country or their independence. Parkes (1993, p. 91), distinguishing between loss and change, which is a part of normal life, and loss which is more major in its implications, refers to 'dangerous life-change events'. These are events which drastically change the way we see the world because many of our previously held assumptions are no longer valid. Our previously 'taken for granted' world may never seem the same again. Nurses and health care professionals are often in contact with people who are traumatised in this way and it helps if they have a framework for understanding how people may experience loss. Not only will this help the professional to feel more confident about working in this area, but it will also enable them to explain to individuals and families what might be happening to them.

Parkes's early work involved research with older people who went suddenly blind. He found that if they were not supported through the initial period of adjustment they failed to develop the skills needed for living with their sight loss. In other words, people needed to mourn their loss first before they could start to re-build their lives. This key finding, supported by subsequent work in this field, has enabled health care professionals to recognise the importance of providing support for people in the early stages of a diagnosis and many of the specialist nursing roles have developed from this premise, for example the clinical nurse specialists in respiratory care, cystic fibrosis, multiple sclerosis, breast care and so on. Some of the early work in breast care suggested that patients receiving specialist nurse intervention following the diagnosis of breast cancer demonstrated less psychiatric morbidity and more beliefs in personal control over health (Maguire *et al.* 1980; Watson *et al.* 1988).

However, there are still many areas within health care that provide no on-going supportive care. This is seen typically within smaller specialties that, for cost reasons, find it difficult to employ such roles due to smaller numbers of patients. Nevertheless, the impact of grief is no less for these patients, and nurses who encounter such patients should be mindful of the need to explore other avenues of support that might be available, such as other counselling services, national support agencies and local support groups as well as engaging the patient's own support network through friends and family.

An example of how supportive care can be provided for dying patients at home and their families is that provided by community nurses and specialist palliative care nurses. A large part of this work will consist in helping the family anticipate the loss and providing support during the period before death occurs. Although there is some debate in the literature about the concept of anticipatory grief – whether or not prior knowledge of impending loss has an impact on someone's grieving process (Weiss 1988; Duke 1998; Costello 1999) – it is nonetheless self-evident that people who go into a crisis with some sort of preparation will adjust to events better than if they had no preparation. A simple way of depicting this as depicted in Figure 5.1 shows the time leading up to an event, the event itself and the period immediately following it.

The event might relate to something stressful which is being anticipated but may not necessarily be a 'dangerous life event', such as death. A simple example might concern an important assessment for which a student has a known submission date.

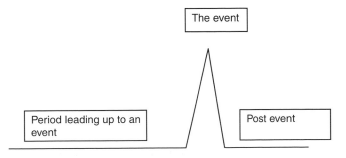

Figure 5.1   Linear representation of the time before and after an event.

The student may prepare for this in a variety of ways, some of which will probably involve 'worry work', reading and preparation, and thinking and talking through aspects of the task with others. If the student had had no warning of the assignment and had to complete it immediately, it is possible that the task would seem too overwhelming and the end result might be a non-submission. In the same way, preparation for an impending loss has the potential to mitigate some of the stresses associated with the uncertainty of loss and enable people to make adjustments. Giving people the opportunity, then, to ask questions, rehearse events, express how they are feeling and seek information will enable them to prepare themselves, however an impossible task that might seem, for what is to come.

Whilst in some circumstances preparation for loss might be helpful, we must remember that the impact of absolute loss can never be imagined. Practical aspects of preparing for loss may include education and preparation for the effects of loss, for example in preparing a patient who is about to lose a limb the nurse might provide information regarding what the scar might look like, or show the patient a prosthetic limb. However, caution must be applied as it is important to recognise the patient who is not ready to acknowledge what is happening and forcing information on the patient at this stage may lead to conflict for the patient and in some circumstances affect the relationship between the nurse and the patient.

If you refer to Figure 5.1 and consider the period of time prior to the death, it is possible for communication to be 'blocked' during that time so that people do not get a chance to prepare or to adjust. One of the ways in which this might happen is if the family does not want any bad news to be discussed with the patient or if the patient himself or herself is in denial about the seriousness of his or her illness. However, it must be remembered that denial is a common response to bad news and loss, for example denial of illness was found to be the most common defence mechanism in response to the diagnosis of cancer (Kortte & Wegener 2004). Freud (1948) described denial as an unconscious defence mechanism that protects the individual from significant trauma. More recent authors have suggested that in some patients denial may even be a conscious decision to maintain privacy and reduce death-anxiety (Zimmerman 2004). Kortte and Wegener (2004) explore the effects of denial within the literature and suggest that whilst denial can be adaptive if it enables the patient to interpret illness in such a way as to maintain hope and optimism, it can have a maladaptive effect on long-term recovery if it is focused on the complete avoidance of the reality of illness.

The drawing in Figure 5.2 was by a patient who was diagnosed with cancer shortly after giving birth to her son. The drawing was done seven years later. At the time of her initial diagnosis she was unable to allow intrusive thoughts of cancer and life-threatening disease into her mind and instead focused on making a future for her son. Several years later, her son was gaining more independence and she was now able to think about the impact of her cancer and seek counselling. The dark clouds in the picture signify her perception of her cancer as blocking the continuation of her life journey. Following the completion of counselling, the picture of the bright sun represents a more positive future. For the health care professional this illustration serves as a reminder that each person will be on his or her own journey in dealing with his or her illness and practitioners need to be guided by each individual as to what is important for each of them at any given stage in

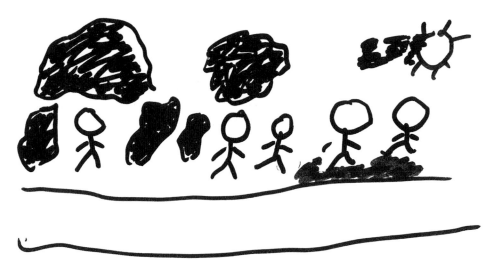

Figure 5.2   The longitudinal journey of grief – a patient's drawing of her cancer journey (reproduced with the patient's permission).

BOX 5.3

The four 'tasks of grieving' (Worden 2003)

Worden, building on the work of earlier theorists like John Bowlby, Colin Murray Parkes and Elizabeth Kubler Ross, suggested that there are 'tasks' which help people to move on in their grief. If these tasks are completed successfully then healing can take place. If they are not completed, the healing may be incomplete. The tasks he outlined were the following:

1. Accept the reality of the loss.
2. Experience the pain of grief.
3. Readjust to an environment in which the deceased is missing.
4. Find an appropriate place for the deceased in the bereaved person's emotional life.

---

that journey. As Sheldon (2004) suggests, however, it is important that professionals do not collude with denial by pretending to share it but that they understand why some patients and families need to maintain it, at least for a time.

Patients may be exhausted by an overwhelming array of emotions which may include anger, denial, fear, shock, helplessness, guilt, regret, searching for reasons and sadness. Being able to be alongside, sometimes in silence, is a real challenge. Care of the family too, during the grieving process, has an important preventive health component as their experiences of the illness and death of their loved one will live on into the future (Monroe & Sheldon 2004). Having an understanding of some of the theories and models of the process of bereavement will help professionals understand what people may be experiencing and how they may be supported through their losses. In this respect, Worden's 'tasks of grieving' (Worden 2003) is a helpful way of conceptualising the way in which people will need to work through the process of mourning towards recovery (Box 5.3).

Activity 5.4

Further reading about loss

Parkes C.M. (1998) Coping with loss. *British Medical Journal* 316: 1521–1524.

This paper is the last in a series of 10 articles dealing with different types of losses. It is written from a practice perspective and focuses on the sorts of losses that may go unrecognised and that health care professionals are particularly well placed to provide support in.

Worden's model can be particularly useful for nurses who may be involved at the time of death in helping relatives 'accept the reality of the death' ('task 1' of Worden's model). Nurses can do this by

- enabling people to be present at the death if they wish to be;
- supporting people who want to spend time with/view the dead body;
- allowing people to express feelings;
- giving opportunity to ask questions;
- giving the death certificate and the dead person's belongings back can be an ideal opportunity for exploring queries and questions;
- clear information-giving. Newly bereaved people can find it very hard to process information;
- letting people know there are choices;
- asking about children, elderly relatives and others who may be 'disadvantaged' from being included in what is going on. See Activity 5.4.

Specific Needs of Children and Other Vulnerable People

If you refer to Figure 5.1 you can see that children who are not kept informed about what is happening in a family where someone is dying may be catapulted into an extremely traumatic event (the death) without any chance to prepare for it or be supported by those closest to them. The same would be true of other vulnerable people who may not have the capacity to seek information – such as people with severe learning difficulties, frail older people or people living with dementia. There is a tendency to want to 'protect' such people by excluding them from information which is distressing, but it is more likely that they will end up being isolated with no opportunity to prepare for significant life changes. If this is the case the likely outcome is that they will experience longer-term bereavement effects (Black 1998).

In a situation of serious illness, children and other vulnerable people need explanations about what is happening in simple, clear language, appropriate to their understanding. There are many books and booklets available to help present concepts and facts to children about serious illness. Children are not good at interpreting euphemisms and so a child who has been told 'we have lost granny' will not necessarily understand that she has died. It is much better to use words like 'dead' and 'has died'. Children generally need concrete experiences and may benefit from the opportunity of seeing a person after death and attending the funeral (see Activity 5.5).

> **Activity 5.5**
>
> **Further reading on communicating with children about loss**
>
> http://www.crusebereavementcare.org.uk
>
> It offers information and advice online and has a series of excellent written material and fact sheets on a variety of matters, for example talking to children about death.
>
> http://www.winstonswish.org.uk
>
> It is a child bereavement charity which helps young people re-adjust to life after the death of a parent or sibling. The site contains information on serious illness, telling the children, preparing for change, the role of schools and so on and also includes a bibliography of helpful books for children and other resources.

Talking about Bad News

No matter how experienced the nurse is in talking about bad news the actual process and delivery of bad news is never easy. One of the important things to recognise is that the patient perception of bad news may be different from that of the professional. Kinghorn (2001, p. 170) describes a patient's relieved response to being told his cancer diagnosis because at least he now knew what he was 'up against'. Sometimes the uncertainty of 'not knowing' can be more difficult to live with than what is known. However, Salander (2002) suggests that it is not uncommon to meet patients who persistently express negative feelings about how they were given bad news and that this has a subsequent effect on their sense of trust.

In terms of patient preferences for information, there is evidence to suggest that most patients want it regardless of the outcome and chances of cure (Arber & Gallagher 2003; Fallowfield & Jenkins 2004). If bad news is communicated badly this may result in resentment, confusion and long-lasting distress, whereas if done well it can assist in acceptance and adjustment (Fallowfield & Jenkins 2004). It is important to remember however that not all patients will want all the information to be given at the same time or at the same level (Davidson & Mills 2005). For some patients denial may be their way of maintaining self-preservation and we must remember that whilst patients have a right to information this should not be translated into a duty to hear it (Baile *et al.* 2000). Equally, we must remember that bad news cannot be translated into good news. Accurate assessment of the patient's need for information is paramount and will include, checking the patient's current understanding of the situation, how they see things at the moment, actively asking the patient if there is anything they would like to know and how much they would wish to be informed about, as well as giving the patient permission to talk about things that concern them.

Assessment should also include assessment of non-verbal behaviour which is likely to convey more information than verbal (Egan 1994). Responding to non-verbal behaviour, maintaining eye contact, assuming an attentive position without physical barriers, active listening, which includes nodding, reflection, facilitating patient disclosure through encouragement, and the demonstration of empathy will further develop the relationship (Ryan *et al.* 2005) and give the professional a clearer understanding of the patient's wishes for information, particularly in relation to bad news.

Whilst in some circumstances it might be more appropriate for the doctor to deliver bad news, multidisciplinary teams should develop protocols on communication identifying all team members' responsibilities within each part of the patient pathway (NICE 2004). In some circumstances, due to the often intimate relationship between the nurse and the patient, the nurse may be considered the most appropriate person. Due to the unique position of nurses who often spend extended periods of time talking to patients, it is not uncommon for the nurse to be specifically asked by the patient to explain the situation to them. Thus, having the skills to convey such information is essential.

Breaking bad news is a complex process and demands expert verbal as well as non-verbal communication skills. Prior to breaking bad news several considerations must be made. First, there should be both time and privacy. Ensuring there is adequate time free from interruption will allow the patient to feel more able to respond and ask questions. For some patients it might be important to have a close family member or friend present. The use of appropriate simple language is also important, avoiding euphemisms and over use of medical terminology, for example, a 'negative' lymph node may be interpreted by the patient as a bad thing rather than the fact that the lymph node was in fact free of disease. Another example of varied interpretation is when the patient is told things are 'progressing', which can of course be interpreted by the patient as things progressing well. A further consideration is ensuring that you have as much information about the patient's medical and psychosocial situation as possible.

During the delivery of bad news it is useful to have a template or protocol to ensure that the information is delivered in a timely, sensitive manner. Key principles to breaking bad news are outlined in Box 5.4.

BOX 5.4

Key principles to breaking bad news. Adapted from Baile *et al.* (2000) and DHSSPS (2004)

- Creating the right environment (privacy, room layout, offering the opportunity to bring a relative or friend).
- Familiarisation with the patient's medical and psychosocial background.
- Checking out the patient's understanding of the situation so far.
- Assessing the patient's need for information, and level of information required (ask the patient how much information he or she would like).
- Give a warning shot prior to imparting the bad news that is 'I am afraid that I have bad news'.
- Ask permission to carry on.
- Provide clear information, using language that the patient can understand.
- Allow some time for the patient to reflect on what has been said.
- Ask the patients how he or she is feeling as well as what he or she is thinking.
- Check with the patients their understanding and whether there is anything they would like to ask.
- Give the patients permission to express their feelings and acknowledge their distress.
- Ask if there is anything that they would want you to do.
- Offer a further consultation at a later date to clarify anything that the patient is unsure of and to check how the patient is coping.
- On completion of the interview ensure that there is appropriate documentation and that key team members are informed.

Activity 5.6

Think about a situation that you have experienced where the patient has recently received bad news. Using the principles outlined in Box 5.4 think about how the news was delivered. What did the nurse or doctor do well? Could anything have been done better? How did the patient respond? How did you feel and how did you respond? Was there any interaction between you and the patient? How did you, or how could you, have helped the patient?

No matter how well rehearsed the delivery of bad news is, it is not only stressful for the patient but also frequently results in an increase in emotion for the nurse. This may be particularly the case if the patient is young or the nurse identifies in some way with the patient. Discussing these feelings with colleagues is important as is the opportunity for supervision. In planning care for the future the nurse must also consider the wider context of care and ensure effective communication with all health professionals who will be involved in the patient's care. The division between acute and secondary care sometimes leaves the patients within a chasm or absence of care, for example when the patient moves from active treatment to palliative care and it is essential that the traditional boundaries of health care provision do not add to the patient's concerns at this time through compartmentalising the patient (Activity 5.6).

Anger

Handling emotions which may follow the delivery of bad news is challenging for the health care professional and one of the most difficult of these is probably anger (Kennedy Sheldon *et al.* 2006). Patients may feel angry that they have become ill as a result of something they have done (or not done) and a common response may be to blame something or someone else. Sometimes it may be the health care professionals who become the focus for the patient or family anger (Kennedy Sheldon *et al.* 2006). However, in the same way as denial, anger may have both positive and negative attributes (Thomas *et al.* 2000). Whilst anger can be immobilising through the constant attention to the past preventing the patient from moving on, it can also be energising, enabling the patients to take greater control over their own health and body.

When patients express anger it is important for the nurse not to become defensive or avoid the person who is angry, but to offer the opportunity to discuss the underlying feelings for anger, allowing the patient to express it (in a non-threatening or violent manner) and to explore ways in which the patients feel their anger might be resolved or used in a positive way.

Conclusion

In this chapter we have looked at some of the challenges of communicating with people facing loss and outlined principles of good practice. We have seen how communication is more effective if in the context of relationship. It is important to remember that relationships develop over time, and are dependent on a number of factors. Expressing an interest in the patient as an individual will encourage a relationship of trust and therefore a willingness to share difficult emotions. Using body language to demonstrate openness, asking open questions and demonstrating empathy with the patient will also help to develop the nurse–patient relationship.

Some patients may experience difficulty in articulating how they feel because the emotions are strange and they are unable to find the right words to describe their emotions. Acknowledging the range of emotions will help patients and families better understand the process of loss and grief and recognise the feelings they are experiencing as normal. Nurses and other professionals may be tempted to try and rescue the patient by saying or doing something to make the patient feel better; yet, it is often impossible to find the right words and this may not be what the patient wants. Offering time to sit with the patient and allowing silence can be just as important in terms of supportive care.

The emotional burden of breaking bad news and caring for patients and families facing loss can be at times extremely demanding, but it can also be immensely rewarding. Health care professionals are often privileged to see the richness of peoples' resources, their generosity and the courage with which they face the unknown. The reverse is also true and health care professionals need the opportunity to transfer and share the burden through discussion with colleagues and supervision. Reflection can also be a way of identifying our own personal difficulties and enabling us to develop strategies for working with difficult emotions in the future. After reading this chapter you may wish to consider your own experience of communicating with people who are seriously ill or facing loss. You will probably also have become aware of areas that you would like to do further reading and reflection on.

References

Alasad J., Ahmad M. (2005) Communication with critically ill patients. *Journal of Advanced Nursing* 50(4): 356–362.

de Araujo T.M.M., da Silva M.J.P. (2004) Communication with dying patients – perception of intensive care unit nurses in Brazil. *Journal of Clinical Nursing* 13(2): 143–149.

Arber A., Gallagher A. (2003) Breaking bad news revisited: the push for negotiated disclosure and changing practice implications. *International Journal of Palliative Nursing* 9: 166–172.

Baile W.F., Buckman R., Lenzi R., Glober G., Beale E.A., Kudelka A.P. (2000) SPIKES: a six-step protocol for delivery bad news – application to the patient with cancer. *Oncologist* 5: 302–311.

Becker R. (2001) 'How will I cope?': psychological aspects of advanced illness. In: *Palliative Nursing: Bringing Comfort and Hope* (eds Kinghorn S., Gamlin R.). Bailliere Tindall, Kidlington, UK.

Black D. (1998) Bereavement in childhood. *British Medical Journal* 316: 931–933.

Chapman K., Abraham C., Jenkins V., Fallowfield L. (2003) Lay understanding of terms used in cancer consultation. *Psycho-oncology* 12: 557–566.

Concise Oxford Dictionary (1991) 8th edn. BCA by arrangement with Oxford University Press, London.

Costello J. (1999) Anticipatory grief: coping with the impending death of a partner. *International Journal of Palliative Nursing* 5(5): 223–231.

Department of Health, Social Services and Public Safety (DHSSPS) (2004) *Breaking Bad News: Regional Guidelines*. DHSSPS Belfast.

Davidson R., Mills M. (2005) Cancer patients' satisfaction with communication, information and quality of care in a UK region. *European Journal of Cancer Care* 14: 83–90.

Duke S. (1998) An exploration of anticipatory grief: the lived experience of people during their spouses' terminal illness and in bereavement. *Journal of Advanced Nursing* 28(4): 829–839.

Dunne K., Sullivan K., Kernohan G. (2005) Palliative care for patients with cancer: district nurses' experiences. *Journal of Advanced Nursing* 50(4): 372–380.

Egan G. (1994) The Skilled Helper. *A Problem Management Approach to Helping*, 5th edn. Brooks/Cole, Belmont, CA.

Fallowfield L., Jenkins V. (2004) Communication sad, bad and difficult news in medicine. *Lancet* 363: 313–319.

Freud S. (1948) *The Ego and the Mechanisms of Defence*. Hogarth, London.

Green A. (1996) An explanatory study of patients memory recall of their stay in an adult intensive therapy unit. *Intensive and Critical Care Nursing* 12: 131–137.

Hack T., Degner L., Parker P. (2005) The communication goals and needs of cancer patients: a review. *Psycho-oncology* 14: 831–845.

Happ M. (2000) Interpretation of nonvocal behaviour and the meaning of voicelessness in critical care. *Social Science and Medicine* 50: 1247–1255.

Harris S., Templeton E. (2001) Who's listening? Experience of women with breast cancer in communicating with physicians. *The Breast Journal* 7(6): 444–449.

Hemsley B., Sigafoos J., Baladin S., Forbes R., Taylor C., Green V., Parmenter T. (2001) Nursing the patient with severe communication impairment. *Journal of Advanced Nursing* 35(6): 827–835.

Heyse-Moore L.H. (1996) On spiritual pain in the dying. *Mortality* 1(3): 297–315.

Humphreys D. (2000) It frightens me. It's personal. Hurry. *Cancer* 89(2): 229–230.

Jarrett N., Payne S. (1995) A selective review of the literature on nurse–patient communication: has the patient's contribution been neglected? *Journal of Advanced Nursing* 22: 72–78.

Kennedy Sheldon L., Barrett R., Ellington L. (2006) Difficult Communication in Nursing. *Journal of Nursing Scholarship* 38(2):141–147.

Kinghorn S. (2001) Communication in advanced illness: challenges and opportunities. In: *Palliative Nursing: Bringing Comfort and Hope* (eds Kinghorn S., Gamlin R.). Bailliere Tindall, Kidlington, UK.

Kortte K.B., Wegener S.T. (2004) Denial of illness in medical rehabilitation populations: theory, research and definition. *Rehabilitation Psychology* 49(3): 187–199.

Levy M. (2001) End of life care in the Intensive Care Unit: can we do better? *Critical Care Medicine* 29(2 supplement): N56–N61.

Maguire P., Tait A., Brooke M., Thomas C., Sellwood R. (1980) Effect of counselling on the psychiatric morbidity associated with mastectomy. *British Medical Journal* 281: 1454–1456.

Maguire P. (1999) Improving communication with cancer patients. *European Journal of Cancer* 35(14): 2058–2069.

Monroe B., Sheldon F. (2004) Psychosocial dimensions of care. In: *Management of Advanced Disease* (eds Sykes N., Edmonds P., Wiles J.). Arnold, London.

NICE (2004) *Improving Supportive and Palliative Care for Adults with Cancer*. National Institute of Clinical Excellence, London.

Nursing and Midwifery Council (NMC) (2007) *Essential Skills Clusters*. NMC Circular 07(2007) Annexe 2, NMC, London.

Parkes C.M. (1993) Bereavement as a psychosocial transition: processes of adaptation to change. In: *Handbook of Bereavement: Theory, Research and Intervention* (eds Stroebe M., Stroebe W., Hansson R.). Cambridge University Press, Cambridge.

Ryan H., Schofield P., Cockburn J., Butow P., Tattersall M., Turner J., Girgis A., Bandaranayake D., Bowman D. (2005) How to recognize and manage psychological distress in cancer patients. *European Journal of Cancer* 14: 7–15.

Salander P. (2002) Bad news from the patient's perspective: an analysis of the written narratives of newly diagnosed cancer patients. *Social Science and Medicine* 55(5): 721–732.

Saunders C. (1965) Watch with me. *Nursing Times*, 26 November.

Sepulveda C., Marlin A., Yoshida T., Ullrich A. (2002) Palliative care: the World Health Organisation's global perspective. *Journal of Pain and Symptom Management* 24(2): 91–96.

Sheldon F. (2004) Communication. In: *Management of Advanced Disease* (eds Sykes N., Edmonds P., Wiles J.). Arnold, London.

Thomas S., Groer M., Davis M., Droppleman P., Mozingo J., Pierce M. (2000) Anger and cancer: an analysis of the linkages. *Cancer Nursing* 23(5): 344–349.

Thorne S., Kuo M., Armstrong E., McPherson G., Harris S., Hislop G. (2005a) 'Being known': patients' perspectives of the dynamics of human connection in cancer care. *Psycho-oncology* 14: 887–898.

Thorne S., Bultz B., Baile W. (2005b) Is there a cost to poor communication in cancer care?: a critical review of the literature. *Psycho-oncology* 14: 875–884.

Watson M.M., Denton S., Baum M., Greer S. (1988) Counselling breast cancer patients: a specialist nurse service. *Counselling Psychology Quarterly* 1: 25–34.

Weiss R. (1988) Is it possible to prepare for trauma? *Journal of Palliative Care* 4(1): 74–76.

Wilkinson S. (1991) Factors that influence how nurses communicate with cancer patients. *Journal of Advanced Nursing* 16: 677–688.

Worden J.W. (2003) *Grief Counselling and Grief Therapy: A Handbook for the Mental Health Practitioner*, 3rd edn. Brunner-Routledge, Hove.

Zimmerman C. (2004) Denial of impending death: a discourse analysis of the palliative care literature. *Social Science and Medicine* 59(8): 1769–1780.

Section 1

Section 2

Organisational Aspects of Care

CHAPTER 6

Value-based Practice

Cathy Sullivan

Introduction

This chapter is concerned with how we develop our practice to see service users as whole people, and how by using a model of health which incorporates spiritual health, mental health, physical health and family health we can contribute to the health and well-being of all those who use our services.

This chapter begins by examining what we mean by value-based practice and value-based decision-making. It explores the meanings of the terms, before asking you what values and qualities are informing your practice, and how these could be used to enhance the care you give to service users. The term value-based practice has developed over the last ten years and is seen as the enhancement of evidenced health care as it integrates the best of evidence-based health care data with the 'perceived quality of life improvement conferred by a healthcare intervention' that is grounded in the service users' perceived value of the intervention given (Brown *et al.* 2005).

The second section considers the factors that encourage and discourage partnership working with service users by exploring ways in which we as health professionals can learn from our experiences and develop reflective skills that will help us to make informed value-based decisions in partnership with our service users. Value-based practice encourages us to trust our intuitions, to value our judgements and to recognise our sensitive qualities and responses. As Seedhouse (2005) states, we are required as health professionals 'to be fully human'.

Lastly, this chapter examines how policy and service development particularly within mental health services is beginning to integrate value-based decision-making into service provision, developing models of care that are service user-centred.

The specific learning outcomes addressed in this chapter, link with the Nursing and Midwifery Council's (NMC 2007) Essential Skills Clusters, and are identified below.

> **Learning outcomes**
>
> By the end of this chapter you will be able to do the following:
>
> - Explain what value-based practice means in health and social care.
> - Describe the key principles to good partnership approaches and processes in value-based practice.
> - Explain the relationship of value-based practice to the Essential Skills Clusters.
> - Begin to apply value-based practice in your work and interactions with service users.

What is Value-based Practice?

Within nursing, several terms are used and applied interchangeably for those who use or come into contact with health or social care services; these include terms like 'patient' or 'client' often depending on the area of practice you are working in. More recently, the term 'service user' has come to be increasingly used, both within Britain and beyond, to describe people on the receiving end of health and social care policies and services. This use of language is contentious. It has come in for criticism as presenting people in passive, consumerist terms. Value-based practice does not suggest that one term is more appropriate than the other, acknowledging the subjective meaning of each. However, many people using services, and others, use the term of themselves; therefore, throughout this chapter in the absence of a more appropriate term, the term 'service user' will be used.

Traditionally, the structure of the NHS has been a paternalistic model of care and practice (Ham 1992). Professionals were perceived to know best how to care for a service user, often making choices on behalf of service users that excluded any concept of participation or input from the service users themselves (Klein 1995). In recent years, the Department of Health (DH) has published a number of policy documents that seek to give service users a sense of choice, reparation and more recently participation in service delivery. A series of papers entitled *Shifting the Balance of Power* (DH 2001a) suggests that a health service which is more responsive to service users will promote services that not only reflect individual preferences but are also more clinically efficient in its use of resources.

Health care and delivery is constantly undergoing change. We are currently undergoing a further change in our response to an increasing need to recognise and respond to the growing complexity of the values involved in health-related decision-making. Value-based practice plays a key role in today's health services by engaging in the experiences of people who use services, and in the experiences of their families/carers. As Robinson (2005) has highlighted, for this to happen we need to engage in discussion with those people who use our services.

This approach requires that all staff working within the health services have an in-depth understanding of social inclusion, placing the people, with their individual values, beliefs and experiences, at the centre of the care process and recognising that the service user perspective is of equal importance to that of the practitioner. The implications for us as health professionals is that we need to develop an understanding of our own beliefs and values in order that we can come to an understanding of both individual and shared values of the service users we meet.

The Joseph Rowntree Foundation report on *Making User Involvement Work* (Branfield *et al.* 2006) highlights that there have been several initiatives that have taken forward both the idea and practice of user involvement. Such movements have included mental health service users, older people, people with learning difficulties, palliative care service users and other groups. It is clear that significant progress has been made in advancing this participatory approach to policy and service delivery. The political agenda of user involvement is clearly pushing this forward. Strategic changes in service delivery have occurred that are clearly 'putting the service user at the centre', 'empowering the public' and 'working in partnership' with people. Many who would traditionally have been seen as unable to participate have become actively involved in trying to improve the support and services that they and others like them receive.

If user involvement is to move beyond the rhetoric of a political agenda, and the user voice is truly to be listened to and become more than representation on committees, we must now, as health professionals, begin to look at our everyday practice and start to ask questions regarding as to how we involve service users in the care being given and explore how their values are informing their choices in the care they receive on a daily basis. The nursing skills within the Care, Compassion and Communication section of the Essential Skills Clusters (NMC 2007) actively encourage this process. Greater engagement with the service users' values is not simply morally beneficial, but it is also contributing to improved health outcomes. The underlying assumption is that if health benefiting decisions are made that respect values as well as the underpinning evidence, following a process in which values have been explored, clarified and balanced, such decisions are more owned and more likely to be acted on.

Evidence-based Practice

As value-based practice is the sister framework that has grown out of the evidence-based movement, it is important that we first explore evidence-based practice so we can apply its principles to value-based practice.

Evidence-based medicine has been defined as 'the conscientious, explicit and judicious use of current best evidence in making decisions about the care of individual patients' (Sackett *et al.* 1996). Since it was brought to prominence by Sackett and colleagues in the 1990s, evidence-based medicine has been developed and used throughout all parts of health care delivery. The term evidence-based medicine has changed to evidence-based health care to reflect the importance of all types of research rather than just the quantitative research methodologies that the original term evidence-based medicine implied.

Evidence-based practice represents a professional, verifiable, service-user-focused alternative to the inherent risks of untested, ritualistic health care; nonetheless, evidence must be proven relevant and reliable before its value and appropriateness for directing health care is accepted (Fitzpatrick 2007; Libberton & Brown 2007). Evidence-based practice therefore involves assessing the methodological

---

BOX 6.1

The classic model for reviewing available evidence

- Clarifying the question for appraisal about the effectiveness of a particular treatment.
- Searching for primary studies that address this question.
- Appraising the quality of these studies in terms of their ability to answer the efficacy question.
- Extracting the data from each proficient study on the outcomes of the treatment in that particular trial.
- Synthesising the data by collating/reviewing the results of all competent clinical trials.
- Disseminating the findings about the overall efficacy of the treatment.
- Strive to do no harm.

---

quality of research evidence to determine if the findings are of use to inform practice (Greenhalgh 2001). It has been defined by Greenhalgh (2001) as the technique of assessing and interpreting evidence by systematically considering its validity, results and relevance. The two key concepts that concern the quality of research are validity and reliability. Validity concerns the extent to which the research measures what it intended to measure. Reliability refers to the consistency of measurement within a study and enables consistent results to be gained (Gerrish & Lacey 2006). If the research is severely flawed in its validity and reliability, then the results are unlikely to be useful in informing future practice. It is, therefore, fundamental that any research study being used to inform/ guide practice must first be assessed for its quality before practical changes take place.

To practise evidence-based practice, it is important to ask questions regarding care. For example, is the 'treatment approach effective?' The next step is to break the question down into a format that is answerable. The evidence is then searched, key literature identified and appraised. The results generate an enhancing knowledge, giving empirically grounded rational decisions (Box 6.1).

Evidence and decision-making

The demand that practice should be evidence based requires that as health professionals we are able to interpret, evaluate and apply published research findings into our work (Gomm *et al.* 2000). However, not all published evidence can be used for making decisions about service user care due to differing quality, validity and credibility. It is, therefore, necessary to assess the quality, importance and applicability of any research evidence that is being consulted to answer a specific clinical question (Craig & Smyth 2002).

Evidence-based practice greatly improves the effectiveness of health care. Once you are familiar with the terminology, are able to differentiate the quality of evidence for interventions, you can apply this to your practice to facilitate delivery of the highest level of care. However, Seedhouse (2005) raises questions as to why do we rate evidence and reason as more important than our emotional powers or see them of little consequence to the care we give?

Seedhouse (2005) uses the analogy of the fictional character Mr Spock the half Vulcan, half human from the Star Trek series, who advocates the use of logic over emotion. Mr Spock believes that all problems and decisions are better solved using logic and reason, and that as humans we must learn to be less emotional. The Vulcan philosophy is that if logic is independent of emotion, then every logical problem-solver will arrive through a process of deduction at the same best decision. In a sense, evidence-based practice asks us to do the same. That is, if all decisions regarding the best treatment approach are based entirely on quality evidence, research results and clinical reason, then rational decision-making in the form of clinical guidelines and policies can be made in the best interests of the service user.

Why is it then that clinical guidance drawn from the available evidence to guide practice by the National Institute for Clinical Excellence (NICE) is not always accepted as the best option for all service users, and why do user groups challenge their outcomes? For example, NICE (2005) advocated that prescribing of the anti-dementia drugs (donepezil, rivastigmine and galantamine) for early-stage Alzheimer's was unclear after undertaking a systematic review of nine randomised controlled trials. The main issue was whether the modest benefits seen in the outcome measures used in the trials would translate into benefits significant to service users. Based on these findings they consequently limited their availability on the National Health Service (NHS), as the logical analysis of available evidence and cost analysis found the drugs to have little benefit to the service user. This decision did not take into account the service user's view of the value of these drugs. Neil Hunt, the Chief Executive of the user group, Alzheimer's Society, challenged this decision stating the following:

> This seems just another example of the NHS failing to take dementia seriously as a medical condition. Despite the fact that these drugs are proven to work, NICE believes that they aren't good value for money. We know they are. The Society has seven years of evidence that proves that these drugs improve the quality of people's lives. NICE seem to think that people with dementia aren't worth spending money on, but how else can you change someone's life for just £2.50 a day? (Hunt 2005)

This is a clear example of where clinical evidence does not take into account the service user's opinion or emotional reactions to the value of intervention. The decision not to prescribe was subsequently challenged and won the Alzheimer's Society the right to appeal the judgement.

Value-based Practice

Value-based practice aims to take evidence-based practice to a higher level (Brown *et al.* 2005). For value-based practice also includes all the service users' 'perceived quality-of-life' variables associated with an intervention, thus allowing a more accurate measure of the overall worth of that intervention to the service user than a decision based solely on a primary evidence-based outcome. This allows the health practitioner to tailor care and deliver higher quality care by giving service users what they value most.

Value-based practice is a framework that aspires to make health care more attentive to the service user as unique individuals. Its aim is to contribute to the decision-making process improving health outcomes by ensuring that decisions are owned by the service user as reflecting their views, concerns and wishes based on their beliefs and values.

How is value measured?

To date, the main evaluation model in looking at value has been based on health economics as a cost–utility analysis, in which the benefits of health care are valued in terms of quality-adjusted life years (QALYs). This approach poses challenges when making decisions for service users based on evaluations of single health care interventions, which inevitably involve judgements about whether the QALYs gained are worthwhile, or, in other words, what is the monetary value of a QALY. Within this model ethical reasoning requires that service user values are normally given in a hypothetical manner often in the form of assertions about 'dignity', 'choices' or 'autonomy' within care, or on most occasions they are more likely to be expressed as wishes, preferences, hopes or fears in relation to a contextual event. This allows values to be represented numerically, so that a mathematical equation can be used to produce an answer to guide our actions.

The total number of QALYs conferred from a health intervention is calculated by adding the following components of a proposed intervention (Brown *et al.* 2005):

(the utility value improvement conferred by the intervention) × (the duration of the treatment benefit during pre-treatment life expectancy) + (the utility value of the post-intervention health state) × (the number of years of life added by the intervention)

The total value conferred by an intervention should then take into account all value gains as well as the value lost due to adverse effects associated with the intervention. The difficulty with this approach is in the subjectivity of the value perception. Undertaking this type of calculation is easy with conventional measurements. Again, Seedhouse (2005) gives us a clear picture of this difficulty, explaining that we can measure a mile, but how do we measure a subjective element like anxiety or fear. No one else can measure my anxiety because they do not have access to it; they can try using an anxiety rating scale but because each of us feels anxiety differently, this means that it is impossible to say objectively that what I experience is or is not fear or anxiety (a sensation that one person thinks of as fearful and anxiety provoking may be pleasurable to another). An example of this would be my experience of Space Mountain at Disneyland Paris – I was petrified and I have the photo to prove it, but the girl in the photo in front of me is laughing and making gestures to the camera. Half a mile is half a mile, what half afraid is, is pretty much anyone's guess, but I in my experience was truly afraid even if others experienced it as pleasure!

This approach therefore tries and fails to put the reasoning back into value-based decision-making, by attempting to bring together findings, approaches and messages. Together they attempt to make it feel that the decisions reached are owned by the service user as reflecting their wishes, concerns and values. However, the challenge for us as health professionals is to take this further, as identity-defining values are often used to contextualise the user voice, but it makes it difficult to identify the personal component in it and challenges us to look for a different model.

Values and beliefs

Much of the work regarding taking this beyond a simple equation into everyday practice has been undertaken in New Zealand where the conflicting values between traditional Maori cultural beliefs and values and Western ethics and values have created new ways of thinking as to how to gain the user voice and where the emphasis is on 'cultural sensitivity' when dealing with service users with no consideration of a power imbalance in the health care setting (Papps 2002). Within nursing practice in New Zealand, this has developed into 'culturally safe' practice which meets the following criterion: actions which recognise and respect and nurture the unique cultural identity of the Maori people and also those of other cultures. The term cultural safety is used to encompass a shift in power to the client and has been defined by the Nursing and Midwifery Council of New Zealand as

> the effective nursing of a person/family from another culture by a nurse who has undertaken a process of reflection on own cultural identity and recognises the impact of the nurse's culture on own practice. Unsafe practice is any action which diminishes, demeans or disempowers the cultural identity and well being of an individual. (Nursing Council of New Zealand, 1992, p. 1, glossary)

Once this transfer of power has occurred the participants of care are true partners and are able to say how they want care to be given, being seen as the experts in their own care. Spence (2005a) highlights this point by explaining that to be culturally safe and value the opinion and views of our service users, we are required to experience ourselves in relation to a person who is 'culturally other'. It requires that we notice the service user as different from us, yet similar to other service users in terms of their need for care. Paradoxically then, it means simultaneously engaging with similarity and difference. However, this approach requires us to provide appropriate responses in relation to individual events which are based on the less measurable dimensions of attitudes, beliefs and values. This requires that all interactions with others are unique, but that the power differential between us will be constant; based on mutual respect. T.S. Eliot reminds us of the relationship between our beliefs and values and our interactions, interpretations and responses. He also describes the inextricable interrelationship of past, present and future development. 'Time past and time future/What might have been and what has been/Point to one end, which is always present' (T.S. Eliot – 'Burnt Norton' 1990). This possibility acknowledges the infinite nature of human understanding. It gives potentialities that are diverse where there is openness to new understandings; however, this requires that we are self-aware (Activity 6.1).

Activity 6.1

Further reading

Try reading some more about this thinking in Seedhouse D. (2006) *Values-based Decision-making for the Caring Professions.* Wiley, Chichester.

Developing Self-awareness and Recognising Our Values

Burns and Bulman (2000) state that being self-awareness is hard to avoid, as self-interest is part of human nature. They argue that developing an honest self-aware-ness is a more complex skill. It is natural to want to see and portray ourselves in a favourable light and this desire, together with our own prejudices and assumptions, can interfere with our ability to objectively look at ourselves. Being honest about oneself therefore requires a degree of self-confidence, as well as personal maturity and the support of others (Burns & Bulman 2000).

Our values are an essential part of who we are as a person. 'Values are closely related to meaning – the meaning of life. The inner meaning of an action, an experience or an attitude gives us our values' (Tschudin 1992, p. 2) It requires us to seek out and recognise our values and ask ourselves the question as to whether we judge our behaviour in terms of what others may believe or in terms of what we 'sense is right for them'? We cannot answer this unless we are aware of who we are and what our beliefs and values are.

Jasper (2003) has identified that we all practice from a belief and values system that has arisen from life experiences and those whom we have encountered, and suggests that personal values and beliefs are founded on the following sources:

- Our religious beliefs and moral up-bringing
- Our ethnic origins
- Our educational opportunities
- Our social class
- The environment in which we grew up
- Our life experiences.

Jasper (2003) stresses that the importance of recognising the uniqueness of our beliefs and values and how these influence our relationship with others, and that these should lie at the heart of our role as health care professionals.

Augustine (Augustine of Hippo, AD 354–430; cited in Thompson *et al.* 2006) said, 'if you wish to know what a man is, ask what he loves'. Our interests also help define who we are, what we strive for and what we are willing to do. Because often our initial feelings are so personal and often transient, they are not a sufficient basis on which to base moral judgements. We clearly need and look for other evidence to base our reasoning and the principles on which we base our moral beliefs and decision-making. Often our comfort in the right choice is evidence-based practice because it is logical (Seedhouse 2005).We also develop a values base and identity that fits with our professional accountability as defined by the NMC

(2008) Code. Nursing is not perceived as value free by the general public, and we are expected to be able to consider the kind and range of everyday ethical issues that we encounter each time we meet a service user and be aware through the process of reflection as to how this is influencing both our personal values system and professional standing.

Thompson *et al.* (2006) support this view that we make moral judgements all the time often in the light of what we consider the best course of action. They argue that we tend to appeal to the 'voice of conscience' or 'intuition', or often just say 'it felt right'. While these expressions have a place in our moral code and are often based on societal codes playing a key role within our decision-making, they are often a refusal to look inwards and identify the underlying reasons as to why we have acted in a particular way.

MacIntyre (1999) tells us of the importance of self-reflection in relation to moral judgement, proposing that to develop as independent 'reasoners' we need to make the transition from accepting what we have been taught by our parents or early role models to making our own decisions about behaviour. He states that it is only when we are able to make independent judgements that we are truly able to become independent of other people's moral codes and are able to undertake a self-appraisal process.

Consider your values in Activity 6.2. This questioning can be an uncomfortable experience. But understanding 'who we are', learning to appreciate and like parts of our values systems as well recognising those parts that may need up-dating, is important. We normally live by values, and if we do not know what they are, it can come as a surprise when we meet and work with others who hold different values systems and can leave us open to making judgements and having prejudices. Barnum (1996) echoes this view and argues that before nurses can fully care for others, they must care for themselves. Connecting in relationship to others also requires that we connect at a deeper level with ourselves.

In a sense we are all spiritual beings and our spirituality informs our humanity. We do not have to be religious to be spiritual though some people root their spirituality in the religious tradition they belong to. But an authentic spirituality takes us out of ourselves and enables us to focus on the needs and rights of others. True compassion is not feeling sorry for others but having an unreserved sense of their inherent worth and dignity.

You will have thought about what you mean by values in completing Activity 6.2. Clarifying our values is important for us as nurses, since to know and appreciate our values system provides a basis for understanding how and why we react to decision-making. Values direct our lives and are unique to each of us. Being aware of our values, and learning to respect them, facilitates living a life with meaning and purpose. Burkhardt and Nathaniel (2001) advocate that this awareness enables us to experience fulfilment and happiness in our work and relationships, with an enormous effect on the way we act, relate to and communicate with our service users and colleagues. If this is then reciprocated by those around us then common respect, approval and acknowledgement is initiated. In this way an awareness of our values will help us throughout our careers in handling difficult situations. Most importantly, failure to do so may mean there is a danger that our professionalism may be comprised (Thompson *et al.* 2006) (Activity 6.3).

Activity 6.2

Try this values exercise

A personal value can be described by a statement that says what is important and significant to you as an individual. Describe three of your own values by completing this sentence:

It is important to me that …

1.

2.

3.

Do your values always guide your actions? Give examples of when they have done and when they have not.

How did you acquire the key values in your life? Identify specific people or situations that have affected your values.

Activity 6.3

Further reading

You will find out more on this area by reading: Part 11 – Developing principled behavior. In: Burkhardt M.A., Nathaniel A.K. (2001) *Ethics & Issues in Contemporary Nursing*. Thomson Delmar Learning, New York.

Values and Reflection

We will all face challenges and experiences that will ask us to look and re-evaluate our beliefs and values. Use of a reflective model such as John's (2000) model of structured reflection which asks us to undertake our learning in an active way by experiencing and testing our theories in practice as well as being reflective (looking inwards at what internal factors were influencing us), and then becoming involved in exploring the theories and evidence is helpful in enabling us to turn experience into learning, making the most of situations we find ourselves in and applying our experiences in new situations (reflexive learning). Using these principles try to complete Activity 6.4 using Case study 6.1.

Boud *et al.* (1985) highlight that the reflective process begins with me returning to or recollecting an event as in Case study 6.1; exploring behaviour, ideas and

---

Activity 6.4

Read Case study 6.1 and then look at these questions

What are the tensions inherent in this scenario?

What enabled the nurse to move from 'wanting to be a million miles away' to knowing Lucy as a person?

How do you think health professionals expect service users to fit into their way of doing things?

Case study 6.1

Looking after Lucy

As a first-year student on my first practice experience, I clearly remember caring for Lucy as she was one of the most testing and thought-provoking people that I met throughout my training.

Lucy had experienced several strokes resulting in atrophy of her limbs and loss of speech. She was unable to sit straight in her bed, there was weakness, and 'twisting' of one side of her face and the paralysis of the right side of her body made her seem vulnerable and totally dependent. She had dribbled her tea down the front of her nightdress, she smelt of urine and I had been asked to give her a wash. But I was frightened and embarrassed; I wanted to be anywhere but here, I really wanted to go home. My mind teemed with questions – Why did I want to be a nurse? How could I care for this woman when I thought she would be better off dead? What could she understand? How would I communicate with her? Was it possible to help without hurting her? I knew I needed to get to know Lucy as a person and to care for her with respect. But it was challenging. How did I know what her wishes and choices might be when she couldn't speak to me?

I explained that I was going to give her a bed bath, talking complete rubbish and focusing on finding her toiletries and a clean nightdress to cover my fear, and hoping she wouldn't notice my flushed face and that my hands were shaking. It took considerable self-determination and resolve to wash her with the respect and dignity I believed she deserved.

Over the rest of my placement, I began to understand her body language and gradually learned what worked and what didn't by her responses. The talking became easier. I found out about Lucy and her family from her daughter, I began to understand Lucy as a person, recognise and interpret Lucy's reactions and realised that I was making choices on her behalf. There was lots of apologising on my part, but by the end of the placement I realised I had come to know her, not as someone to be frightened of, but as a person with her own needs and rights.

Source: Adapted from Spence (2005b).

feelings with the intention of unpacking and identifying all the emotions, ideas, decisions and actions that were part of the experience. It is important to recognise 'obstructing' feelings, often those aspects of my recollection which were embarrassing or awkward (Boud *et al.* 1985) – 'did I really think maybe Lucy would be better dead'. To make my practice better and to connect with Lucy as a person, I needed to identify what made things embarrassing for me and overcome that feeling by being prepared to share the experience openly with others. Accepting that my prejudice exists allows me to challenge and up-date my beliefs about Lucy. Reflective practice does involve a degree of self-honesty and without this understanding we miss the real opportunity to learn about ourselves. Increasing your self-awareness and ability to be self-critical of your feelings will allow you to meet service users as people and be able to respect and listen to their views. To find out more about self-awareness see Chapter 1, particularly the section on Self-awareness.

Frequently, health care professionals operate from a significantly different viewpoint from the service user. When this happens, practitioners react differently according to their own beliefs and values. The resulting conflict can be both upsetting and baffling for everyone. It may be hard to understand how equally concerned parties can have opposing views. Seedhouse (2005) argues that this is a naive observation, to believe a view can be seen as simply right or wrong. One person's positive values may be another person's negative values, and notions such as 'integrity', 'public interest' and 'excellence' are open to wide interpretation. The idea that we can practice health care which ignores the way the service users measure and define themselves as people is unrealistic and inappropriate. People are still prepared to die in order to maintain their culture, religion, beliefs and values. It is not the place of the health professional to attempt to deny these because they require our services, however altruistic the rationale may be.

The Principles of Value-based Practice

With a growing sense of self-awareness, we can now be more effective in enabling service users to identify their own values system. Aiding them to clearly express their values is important, because a lack of clarity about values in either party may result in inconsistency, confusion, misunderstanding and inadequate decision-making. Burkhardt and Nathaniel (2001) note that this is important as the ability to make informed choices can help the process of informed consent, and as we hand the power of decision-making back to the service users allowing them to be self-governing they, like us, have a right to more than just facts, evidence and information to develop a plan of action. They need the opportunity to discuss and express their values. This partnership working may help prevent harmful consequences related to not addressing differences in values between service users and providers (Figure 6.1).

The model for value-based practice in Figure 6.1 helps us understand this process. It emphasises that the service user sits at the centre of all interventions and that the health professional has a professional responsibility to engage with that person using his or her knowledge of self. Burkhardt and Nathaniel (2001)

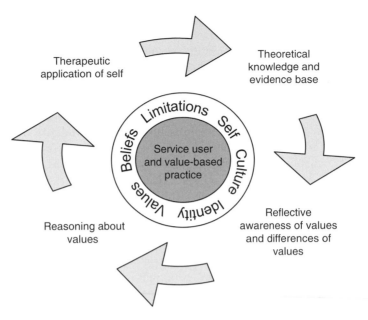

Figure 6.1 A framework for value-based practice (courtesy of Lennon R., Sullivan C. 2007).

strongly emphasise that it is important to remember throughout this process that no one set of values is appropriate for everyone. It is important therefore that we seek values clarification and gain different insights for different service users. Engaging in this process of values clarification promotes a closer fit between the central circle that holds the clients and the surrounding ring enabling us to 'walk in the shoes' of the service user creating sincerity within the professional relationship. This professional sincerity refers to and consists of adherence to the moral norms and professional accountability highlighted within the ring. Individual reflection and discussion with another person or small group can help to ensure we remain sincere and open within these moral norms. Using the skills given in the Care, Compassion and Communication section of the Essential Skills Clusters (NMC 2007) can be a useful tool to undertake this exploration as they each include a statement of service user expectation.

Expanding on Figure 6.1, the four skills areas of value-based practice circling this professional relationship are concerned with the following.

Reflective awareness of values and of differences of values, including

- an awareness of their own emotional state and responses, ensuring these are appropriate to the situation
- an awareness of the emotional state and responses of the service user, incorporating such awareness into their understanding and management of their care
- an awareness of the emotional state and responses of others (for example, colleagues and/or other professional and user groups), in order to develop effective collaborative relationships
- a willingness to take issues to supervision, or to work on them effectively using reflective techniques

Section 2

Reasoning about values: This requires that we have a moral and open dialogue about the intervention in that we are required to work effectively as decision-makers with the service user in a way that recognises cultural safety. It involves the process of placing values within the differing states of external reality, for example, the policies and guidelines required by clinical governance as well as the internal state that is the emotional value placed on the intervention by the service user, taking into account the social and cultural worlds in which they live. Baxter (2001) describes the key components of cultural competence as the following:

- Acceptance of differences as normal, and only to be expected, for human beings.
- Acceptance of the inherent right of all residents in a society to identify as part of the society and acceptance of the resultant changes.

Therapeutic application of self through communication and professional relationship with the service user is crucial for understanding and developing good interpersonal skills and building therapeutic relationships with service users (Bulman & Schutz 2004). Use of therapeutic self occurs when we are able to consciously learn to use ourselves in interactions with others. This then allows the following:

The application of the underpinning theoretical knowledge and relevant evidence base. Burnard (2002) highlights that being self-aware allows us to select therapeutic interventions from a range of options so that the service user benefits more completely. If we are blind to ourselves, we are also blind to our choices. We are blind, then, to caring and therapeutic choices that we could make on behalf of our service users.

An important tool to aid this process is Fulford's (2004) thought-provoking framework of questions which can be applied throughout each skills stage within the cycle for the development of effective value-based decision-making system for practice (Box 6.2, Activities 6.5 and 6.6).

Policy and Practice

A range of health and social care literature and policy guidance, have, over the last ten years, advocated service user and carer involvement in care and decisions about their treatment as well as involvement in the training and education of health professionals. Two of these papers gave a clear starting point to the view that the public should participate in decisions and policies that affect their health and shape health services. First, the NHS Plan ensured that service users and public had a greater say in the NHS (DH 2000). There was clear direction on involving service users and the public in health care, and it set out proposals to introduce Patient Advice and Liaison Services and a Patient Forum in every Trust (DH 2001b). This focus was developed further within Shifting the Balance of Power – the next steps (DH 2001a) by beginning the process of modernising the NHS work force and developing practitioners able to work in partnership with service users and starting to devolve power closer to service users. These papers highlighted the importance

BOX 6.2

Ten principles to develop value-based practice skills (adapted from Fulford 2004)

Fulford gives us ten principles to develop value-based practice skills to enable us to apply value-based practice in each interaction with service users:

Practice skills

- *Awareness*: ensuring you are aware of the values that may play a part in a particular situation
- *Reasoning*: using values as part of your decision-making process to determine 'what is right'
- *Knowledge*: know about values and facts that are relevant to your situation
- *Communication*: using communication skills to resolve conflicts/complexity.

Models of service delivery

- *User centred*: considering the service user's values as the first priority in a given decision
- *Multidisciplinary*: using a balance of perspectives to resolve conflicts

Value-based practice and evidence-based practice

- *The 'Two Feet' principle*: all decisions are based on facts and values; evidence-based practice and value-based practice therefore work together
- *The 'Squeaky Wheel' principle*: values should be involved in all situations and not just be noticed if there is a problem or complex decision to be taken
- *Science and values*: increasing scientific knowledge and evidence-based practice creates choices in health care; this can lead to wider differences in values

Partnership

- *Partnership*: within value-based practice it is important that decisions are taken by service users working in partnership with providers of care.

Source: Table from Fulford K.W.M. (2004). Ten principles of values based medicine. In: *The Philosophy of Psychiatry: A Companion* (ed. Radden J.). Oxford University Press, New York, pp. 206–234; adapted from the table of Fulford K.W.M. *Essentials of Values-based Medicine*, Cambridge University Press, Cambridge (forthcoming).

Activity 6.5

Further reading

If you would like to know more about this framework read: Fulford K.W.M. (2004) Ten Principles of Values Based Medicine. In: *The Philosophy of Psychiatry: A Companion* (ed. Radden J.). Oxford University Press, New York.

Activity 6.6

Using Fulford's (2004) framework, think about the value diversity within a health care setting you have worked in or visited recently. How does it ensure that positive behaviour is demonstrated towards service users?

It may be helpful to consider the following points:

- Does the area identify the impact of different cultures, values and choices upon the delivery of health care provision?
- Does the area understand, respect and value all factors contributing to a positive experience of receiving health care for service users and carers?
- How does working collaboratively with the multi-professional health and social care team improve the service user journey?

---

of the user values, driving integrated care initiatives and promoting partnership working. Whilst later papers gave us clear Government policy to drive this further forward, *Creating a Patient Led NHS* (DH 2005), recognised that becoming truly service-user led would require more than just changes in systems. There needed to be changes in how people behave and changes in culture where everything should be measured by its impact on service users and the benefits to service user health. *The Expert Patients Programme* (DH 2001b) looked directly at chronic conditions and advocated the development of programmes to develop the confidence and motivation of the service user to use their own skills, information and professional services to take effective control over living with a chronic condition.

Hopefully, you now feel ready to start applying the ideas in this chapter to your own practice. Start looking for examples of how value-based practice underpins policy in your area of nursing and then try Activity 6.7.

Many of the ideas underpinning the essential skills clusters are not new. They are based on self-help, empowerment and advocacy. It provides a challenge to traditional notions of professional power and expertise which dominated paternalistic health services for many years. This means that skills are embedded within practice in a way that is enabling service users and carers to deal with and manage their own health promotion or problems and to keep a sense of hope for the future. This can mean enabling them to find a way of life that is rewarding to them whether or not they continue to have health problems.

Conclusion

As health professionals we are subject to performance targets, outcomes and the successful delivery of them. We are part of ongoing professional development and appraisal programmes. We live within constraining and sometimes reducing budgets. All this in itself creates its own challenges, demands and tensions. This could lead us to believe that time to listen to and learn from service users is a luxury we cannot afford on a day-to-day basis. Yet value-based practice is not a threat to our professional skills and expertise but integral to it and its development. The more open and honest we are to the values that inform who we are, the more open and sensitive we may become to the values and cultural background of our service users.

Activity 6.7

Identify one of the following strategies or policies that is of interest to you and will most help to inform your practice and using Fulford's (2004) ten pointers to good process in value-based practice evaluate the values base of your chosen strategy or policy. Note your reasons for why you feel these have been achieved and see if you can make a link between the pointers you identify and one or more of the Essential Skills Clusters (NMC 2007).

Every Child Matters (DH 2003) published alongside the Government's response to Lord Laming's Report into the death of Victoria Climbié, proposes a range of measures to reform and improve children's care. The aim is not only to protect children, but also go beyond and maximise the opportunities open to young people to improve their life chances and fulfil their potential.

The Ten Essential Shared Capabilities Framework (DH 2004) provides a set of key of value-based practice skills that mental health nurses should demonstrate when working with service users. These were developed through consultation with service users, carers, managers, academicians and practitioners. To facilitate this process, a number of focus groups were held across England in order to sample opinion and seek feedback. In the main, they have what might be termed an 'outward focus' and are explicitly and deliberately centred upon the needs of service users and carers.

The Expert Patient – A New Approach to Chronic Disease Management for the 21st Century (DH 2001b). With an ageing population and people living longer, there is an increased risk of long-term chronic conditions such as heart disease, stroke, cancer, arthritis, diabetes mellitus, mental illness, asthma and other conditions. As a result, the predominant disease pattern is one of chronic or long-term illness rather than acute disease. This policy explores how we can work as partners with service users.

Valuing People: A New Strategy for Learning Disability for the 21st Century (DH 2001c) – this strategy sets out the Government's proposals for improving the lives of people with learning disabilities and their families and carers, based on recognition of their rights as citizens, social inclusion in local communities, choice in their daily lives and real opportunities to be independent.

Service users, their families and carers can come to us with a sense of fear and anxiety as to what lies ahead of them. By engaging with them, learning about 'who they are' alongside bringing our professional expertise to their health care, we are affording them the dignity and respect which is rightly theirs. For, as Antoine Saint-Exupery reflects in his story of *The Little Prince*, it is through the heart and not the eyes that we see clearly (De Saint-Exupery, 1995 edition, p. 82).

References

Barnum B. (1996) *Spirituality in Nursing – from Tradition to New Age*. Springer, New York.

Baxter C. (2001) *Managing Diversity and Inequality in Health Care*. Bailliere Tindell, London.

Boud D., Keogh R., Walker D. (1985) *Reflection: Turning Experience into Learning*. Routledge Falmer, London.

Branfield F., Andrews E.J., Chambers P., Staddon P., Wise G., Williams-Findley B. (2006) *Making User Involvement Work – Supporting Service User Networking and Knowledge*. Joseph Rowntree Foundation, York.

Brown M.M., Brown G.C., Sanjay S. (2005) *Evidence-based to Values-based Medicine*. American Medical Association, New York.

Bulman C., Schutz S. (2004) *Reflective Practice in Nursing*, 3rd edn. Blackwell, Oxford.

Burkhardt M.A., Nathaniel A.K. (2001) *Ethics and Issues in Contemporary Nursing*, 2nd edn. Thomson Delmar Learning, New York.

Burnard P. (2002) *Learning Human Skills: An Experiential and Reflective Guide for Nurses and Health Care Professionals*, 4th edn. Butterworth Heinemann, Oxford.

Burns S., Bulman C. (2000) *Reflective Practice in Nursing: The Growth of the Professional Practitioner*. Blackwell Science, Oxford.

Craig J.V., Smyth R.L. (eds) (2002) *The Evidence-based Practice Manual for Nurses*. Churchill Livingstone, Edinburgh.

Department of Health (DH) (2000) *The NHS Plan: A Summary*. The Stationary Office, London.

Department of Health (DH) (2001a) *Shifting the Balance of Power within the NHS*. The Stationary Office, London.

Department of Health (DH) (2001b) *The Expert Patients Programme*. The Stationary Office, London.

Department of Health (DH) (2001c) *Valuing People: A New Strategy for Learning Disability for the 21st Century*. The Stationary Office, London.

Department of Health (DH) (2003) *Every Child Matters*. The Stationary Office, London.

Department of Health (DH) (2004) *The Ten Essential Shared Capabilities – A Framework for the Whole of the Mental Health Workforce*. The Stationary Office, London.

Department of Health (DH) (2005) *Creating a Patient Led NHS*. The Stationary Office: London

De Saint-Exupery (1995 edition) *The Little Prince*. Wordsworth Editions Limited, Ware, Hertfordshire.

Eliot T.S. (1990) *The Complete Poems and Plays*. Faber and Faber, London.

Fitzpatrick J. (2007) Finding the research for evidence-based practice: part one: the development of EBP. *Nursing Times* 103(17): 32–33.

Fulford K.W.M. (2004) Ten principles of values based medicine. In: *The Philosophy of Psychiatry: A Companion* (ed. Radden J.). Oxford University Press, New York, pp. 206–234.

Gerrish K., Lacey A. (eds) (2006) *The Research Process in Nursing*, 5th edn. Blackwell Science, Oxford.

Gomm R., Hammersley M., Foster P. (eds) (2000) *Case Study Method*. Sage, London.

Greenhalgh T. (2001) *How to Read a Paper*. BMJ Publishing Group, London.

Ham C. (1992) *Health Policy in Britain: The Politics and Organisation of the National Health Service*. Macmillan, Basingstoke.

Hunt N. (2005) *Dementia Drugs Work but are too Expensive for the NHS*. Alzheimer's Society, available at http://www.alzheimers.org.uk/site/scripts/press_article.php?articleID=162 (accessed 30/7/2008).

Jasper M. (2003) *Beginning Reflective Practice*. Nelson Thomas Ltd, Cheltenham.

Johns C. (2000) *Becoming a Reflective Practitioner. A Reflective and Holistic Approach to Clinical Nursing, Practice Development and Clinical Supervision*. Blackwell Science, Oxford.

Klein R. (1995) *The New Politics of the NHS*. Longman, London.

Lennon R., Sullivan C. (2007) *Model for Values Based Practice* (unpublished). Adapted from Lennon R., Sullivan C., Carpenter D. (2006) You can't do it all at a distance: what happened to the face of nursing? Poster presentation National Mental Health Nursing Conference, Cambridge.

Libberton P., Brown J. (2007) Critique and Appraisal of the Evidence. In: *Principles of Professional Studies in Nursing* (eds Brown J., Libberton P.). Palgrave, Basingstoke.

MacIntyre A. (1999) *Dependent Rational Animals: Why Human Beings Need Virtues*. Gerald Duckworth, London.

National Institute for Clinical Excellence (NICE) (2005) *Alzheimer's Disease – Donepezil, Galantamine, Rivastigmine and Memantine* (review). Stationary Office, London.

Nursing and Midwifery Council (NMC) (2007) *Essential Skills Clusters*. NMC Circular 07(2007) Annexe 2, NMC, London.

Nursing and Midwifery Council (NMC) (2008) *The Code: Standards of Conduct, Performance and Ethics for Nurses and Midwives*. Nursing and Midwifery Council, London.

Nursing Council of New Zealand (1992) *Guidelines for the Cultural Safety Component in the Nursing and Midwifery Education*. Nursing Council of New Zealand, Wellington.

Papps E. (2002) Cultural safety: what is the question? In: *Nursing in New Zealand: Critical Issues, Different Perspectives* (ed. Papps E.). Pearson Education, Auckland.

Robinson S.T. (2005) *Tohunga – The Revival, Ancient Knowledge for the Modern Era*. Reed , Auckland.

Sackett D.L., Rosenberg W.M.C., Gray J.A.M., Haynes R.B., Richardson W.S. (1996) Evidence based medicine: what it is and what it isn't: It's about integrating individual clinical expertise and the best external evidence. *British Medical Journal* 312(7023): 71–72.

Seedhouse D. (2005) *Values-based Decision-making for the Caring Professions*. Wiley, Chichester.

Spence D.G. (2005a) Hermeneutic notions augment cultural safety education. *Journal of Nursing Education* 44(9): 409–414.

Spence D.G. (2005b) Exploring prejudice, understanding paradox and working towards new possibilities. In: *Cultural Safety in Aotearoa New Zealand* (ed. Wepa D.). Pearson Education, Auckland.

Thompson I.E., Melia K.M., Boyd K.M., Horsburgh D. (2006) *Nursing Ethics*, 5th edn. Churchill Livingstone, Edinburgh.

Tschudin V. (1992) *Values*. Bailliere Tindall, London.

Section 2

CHAPTER 7

Management of Care and Self

Robert Henry Carter

Introduction

The purpose of this chapter is to help you to understand what it means when nurses talk about the *Management of Care and Self*. Amongst all of the changes that have occurred within the development of nurse education curricula over recent years at both pre- and post-qualified levels is the constant that, broadly speaking, the 'management of care' continues to enjoy a high profile in being deemed an essential part of educational provision. Whilst it could be tempting to assume that this represents a current trend or fashion which might soon be replaced with some other equally or more deserving subject to focus on, the continued emphasis and priority that educational commissioners place on the topic is testament to the relevance of this area of study and practice. This means that the subject is not only of interest to those who are about to enter their respective part of the nursing register, but that it will continue to feature in being a major part of their educational development throughout their careers.

In essence, just as being a technically competent practitioner is incumbent on the individual nurse as a means of maintaining his or her professional standing, equally so, the way in which nurses are able to demonstrate and develop their management skills, is increasingly an expectation that the nurse has to achieve. Nowhere is such an expectation better articulated than in the relatively recent publication by the NMC of the Essential Skills Clusters criteria which expresses requirements for entry to the nurse's respective branch and part of the register. In selecting just one of the criteria to justify the importance of the subject area, the need to demonstrate managerial skills competently becomes obvious. Under the heading of 'Organisational Aspects of Care' for example, patients and clients are asked to trust newly registered nurses to 'be confident in their own role within the multi-disciplinary/multi-agency team and to inspire confidence in others' (NMC 2007, p. 13).

The specific learning outcomes addressed in this chapter link with the Nursing and Midwifery Council's (NMC 2007) Essential Skills Clusters, and are identified below.

> **Learning outcomes**
>
> By the end of this chapter you will be able to do the following:
>
> - Understand the rationale for why the 'management of care and self' is a key area in which professional nurses need to develop their skills and knowledge.
> - Consider the roles that managers have to play.
> - Use Mintzberg's ten key roles for managers as a theoretical framework, and consider some ways in which nurses can develop their management skills.

Managing Health Care

There are of course lots of different types of managers in health and social care environments, and it is all too easy to assume that the image of a modern-day health service manager is someone dressed in a smart business suit who operates some distance away from all clinical or caring activity. Whilst it is true that within a sophisticated service such as the National Health Service (NHS) the traditional picture of the professional manager does exist, it is also the case that the bulk of day-to-day managerial activities and decisions are indeed undertaken by staff who do not necessarily have the title 'manager' or the practice of 'management' recorded in their job description. As the largest professional grouping within the health service is nursing, the managerial activities are more likely to include the type of duties which are associated with direct patient and client care. Nurses, then, have to manage at the direct interface of service provision, and their ability to perform well in this area will have a profound effect on patient/client care and leave a lasting impression on the service user and his or her family.

Over recent years, the opportunities for nurses to get involved in management activities have increased and there is now a stated set of expectations which have been set out within *The NHS Plan* (Department of Health (DH) 2000) for nurses to aspire to. Referred to by the Chief Nursing Officer as the 'ten key roles for nurses', they are outlined in Box 7.1.

> **BOX 7.1**
>
> **Ten key roles for nurses (DH 2000)**
>
> - To order diagnostic investigations such as pathology test and X-rays
> - To make and receive referrals direct, for example, to a therapist or a pain consultant
> - To admit and discharge patients for specified conditions and within agreed protocols
> - To manage patient case loads, for example, in areas such as diabetes
> - To run clinics, for example, in ophthalmology
> - To prescribe medicines and treatments
> - To carry out a wide range of resuscitation procedures including defibrillation
> - To perform minor surgery and outpatient procedures
> - To triage patients using the latest IT to the most appropriate health professional
> - To take a lead in the way local health services are organised and in the way they are run.

These roles represent real opportunities for nurses to engage and are consistent with an environment that recognises the need for professionals to assume greater amounts of autonomy whilst retaining the need to be accountable, as set out in the Nursing and Midwifery Council's Code (NMC 2008). This overall set of expectations indicating that nurses need to take on greater responsibility has not been enforced on the profession without its consent. Even if one goes back to 1992, the then United Kingdom Central Council for Nursing, Midwifery and Health Visiting (UKCC) published its influential *Scope of Professional Practice* (UKCC 1992) document which signified that nurses would assume extra responsibility. Nurses then have a good deal more scope for exercising their own judgement concerning how patient/client care is performed as long as this does not compromise care and safety and the NMC Code (NMC 2008) is not contravened (Humphris & Masterton 2000). Since then, there have been a whole raft of initiatives which, although taking a lead from the ten key roles mentioned above, have produced a momentum whereby role change in the shape of extended and advanced practice roles has become the norm. Although this in part has been in response to pragmatic considerations concerning, for example, complying with junior medical staff employment issues, in particular the EU Working Time Directive (EU 1993), equally there has been a genuine demand created by the changing shape and nature of health and social care within the United Kingdom.

Delivering health care in the future

In January 2008 the UK Prime Minister, Gordon Brown, gave a speech to a range of health professionals in London outlining his vision for the future of health care in this country. Consistent with much of the rhetoric that has been coming from the DH and policy analysts, the Prime Minister stated that the 'NHS of the future will do more than treat patients who are ill – it will be an NHS offering prevention as well' (*The Guardian* 2008). Although in practical terms this has been interpreted quite rightly as suggesting the necessity for more testing and screening for conditions like diabetes and kidney disorders, the implication also is that such preventative measures will take place in locations which are much more convenient to the general public and will increasingly be carried out by health care professionals other than doctors. Not surprisingly, nurses and particularly those who operate in community settings will find themselves in the 'front-line' when it comes to delivering and managing services. As the focus of health care is shifting from what Hunter (2003) has referred to as the 'downstream agenda' where treatment of illness was the major preoccupation, to the 'upstream agenda' with its emphasis on prevention and management of conditions, then arguably nurses once again find themselves in a very convenient position to take advantage of the opportunities that will exist for them in working within a model that is underpinned by the caring philosophy more traditionally associated with the profession.

That is not to say that the medical model, whereby cure and treatment largely determined by clinical intervention, has lost its relevance. Acute services will continue to demand the highly skilled technical nurse, but the realisation that people are increasingly living longer and with this may develop more complex chronic conditions, calls for a different set of skills. Such an approach to the management of long-term conditions is well illustrated by the introduction of specific roles within nursing such as those used by the much heralded introduction of Community Matrons. When one adds to this further examples of initiatives that demonstrate nurses acting in more advanced and proactive roles such as specialist diabetes nurses running their own clinics, those who work in NHS Walk In Centres and for services such as NHS Direct, then it is plain to see that these new sets of responsibilities call for a greater awareness about not only how to manage self but increasingly how to manage the work of others who have a role to play in delivering the service to the patient/client.

It is these final points which will be the focus of this chapter. This recognises that much of the literature around management for nurses seems to cater for the needs of those who have moved into what is often referred to as an administrating position whereby management is concerned with the overall provision of services at quite a strategic level. Nurses who work in the front line also have to demonstrate considerable knowledge and skills in their management practice. In this sense, the ability to perform efficiently and effectively as a manager of care will serve the most important beneficiary of your nursing practice – the patient/client.

The Roles and Activities of Managers – The Theoretical Viewpoint

Before attempting to embark on a review of the types of managerial activities nurses require in demonstrating competency in the management of care, it might be useful to consider some generic roles and elements that comprise what managers actually do. One of the original and most influential views of management is the identification that it can be viewed as a *process* of activities (Fayol 1949) which when put together represents a logical and systematic approach to what the purpose of management is. This so-called *classical* view comprises of the functions of planning, organising, commanding, co-ordinating and controlling. Although it is perhaps uncomfortable to use terms such as 'commanding' in this day and age, the basic underlying assumptions behind this process-orientated approach are still recognised for their relevance today, and one can see the influence of such a model within the well-established 'nursing process' with its emphasis on assessment, diagnosis, planning, implementation and evaluation (Wilkinson 2007).

However, even though it might be easy to recognise a logical and systematic rationale for the activities that should guide the practice of management, this still does little to help us in identifying exactly what managers do, and without this it becomes difficult to establish what skills and competencies a good functional manager needs to acquire. Over the years a good deal of work and research has been carried out in order to establish this very thing. Two of the most well-known attempts to do this are provided by Hales (1993) and Mintzberg (1998). Hales (1993) has summarised what he sees as similar elements existing within management work and this was taken from studies which broadly covered a period of approximately 30 years. These included acting as figurehead or leader, monitoring and disseminating information, negotiating with staff, dealing with disruptions, allocating resources, directing others, liaison activities, innovating and planning. Hales (1993) also went on to state that all of these activities were carried out

---

BOX 7.2

Key roles (Handy 1999)

Interpersonal or Leading
- Figurehead – displaying formal and symbolic authority
- Leader – setting an example for others to follow in promoting the interests of the organisation
- Liaison – developing relationships within and outside of the organisation.

Informational or Administrating
- Monitoring – seeking information about what is going on
- Dissemination – passing on such information which may not only be factual but also reflect values and feelings
- Spokesperson – articulating information not only for those inside the organisation but also to the general public.

Decisional or Fixing
- Entrepreneur – seeking out opportunities and developing ways to improve things
- Disturbance handler – making the best of events which are unscheduled and difficult to predict
- Resource allocation – placing resources where they are likely to have the greatest effect
- Negotiation – achieving the best outcomes internally with staff members and also externally with suppliers and patients/clients.

---

within an environment which was characterised by uncertainty, for example management work is of a fragmented and eclectic nature where one has to react to quickly changing events. In complementing the work of Hales (1993), Mintzberg (1998) was interested in why managers do what they do and he answered this by suggesting that they fulfil certain key roles. He categorised these into three distinct groups which are referred to as interpersonal, informational and decisional. It may be easier to think of these in the terms Handy (1999) uses – leading, administrating and fixing (Box 7.2).

Mintzberg's (1998) roles are a very useful means by which we can categorise what and why managers do what they do, and it is this thematic framework which will be used in terms of locating the key areas whereby managers of care need to develop this aspect of their nursing practice. Before we go on to examine such activities in more detail, it is worth pointing out that all managers do of course work within limitations that will affect their ability in carrying out their management practice. This is to be expected across all organisational life. Organisations are very complex and health and social care organisations are no exception to this rule. A good way of reminding us of the ever-present phenomenon of working to such limitations is provided by some concepts developed by Stewart (1982). Much of her work is derived from her experiences of the British health care service and so it is of particular relevance to us here. Stewart (1982) suggested that one can analyse the job of a manager in terms of three criteria which are *demands, constraints and choices*.

The *demands* refers to what you must do in order to carry out your job, *constraints* are about what you are not allowed to do, whilst *choices* refer to the freedom that you have to do things as you wish. As was stated in the introduction to this chapter, the acquisition of greater autonomy and responsibility that some nurses now enjoy has particular relevance for this final element of choice identified by Stewart. As a means of illustrating each of these elements, a demand might be one which is self-imposed such as your own high standard of care you feel needs to be given to a patient/client. A constraint might be the physical location and environment in which you have to practice. The choices could be the range of skills which you have that might limit how you are able to treat a patient/client (Activity 7.1).

Activity 7.1

Think of an area of your nursing practice and list the demands, constraints and choices that you have to work within in order to deliver and manage that care effectively? You could represent this diagrammatically with labels using the diagram below to indicate the level and extent of demands, constraints and choices.

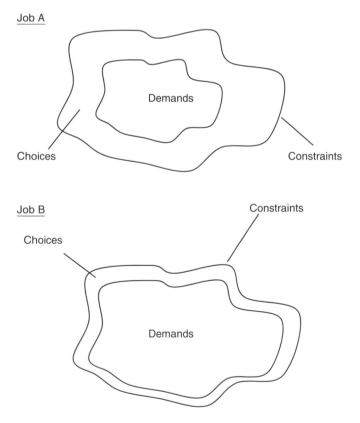

Does your job resemble Job A or is it more like Job B?

Source: Adapted from Stewart (1982) (replicated with kind permission of R. Stewart).

Interpersonal or Leading Roles

When student nurses become registered professionals, their peers, colleagues and patients/clients view them in a completely different light. Not only do the symbols physically change for nurses who work in a setting where status is so obviously connected to uniform, but the expectations of those around change accordingly. To an extent this seems somewhat unfair as the skills and knowledge levels of a newly qualified nurse cannot possibly be transformed overnight. There does, however, have to be a fairly rapid acceptance on behalf of the nurse that his or her professional status has increased dramatically and that part of the responsibilities that will need to accompany this is the requirement to promote himself or herself as a competent and assured professional.

Developing your role as a 'figurehead'

One particular approach to help promote the role of figurehead is strongly associated with the idea of setting a good example in terms of one's values and approach to practice. The discipline of the work place is of course quite contrasting to that of being a full-time student and it is important to quickly accept and conform early on to the expectations of how a professional should behave. There are, of course, clear things one can do right from the start in terms of a smart professional appearance and good time-keeping to name but two. However, there also needs to be a recognition that nurses are like so many other workers in health and social care, which is that they are essentially public servants. Following concerns expressed by many people, and the exploits of some particularly high-profile public servants in the past, that they were in fact putting their own personal interests before the people they were appointed to serve, Lord Nolan was commissioned to carry out a review of standards in public life and make some recommendations. Whilst his findings initially can be seen as being directed to those who hold high public office, many of the values expressed in these principles can also be applied to anyone who has a level of responsibility in delivering a public service, and of course nurses are very applicable here. The Nolan Committee (1996) therefore stressed values which appear to go to the heart of good nursing care and should be present when as a manager of care one is considering developing their self-image and standing. The recommendations, for example, stressed the need to demonstrate selflessness, integrity, accountability and honesty. This can be applied not only to how one approaches relationships with patients/clients, but it should also be all encompassing in terms of the professional's relationship with colleagues.

Developing your role as a 'leader'

Although it might be unreasonable at the very early stages of a nurse's career to expect them to develop the necessary qualities associated with becoming an effective leader, there is an increasingly important recognition that 'leadership' has gained a huge amount of prominence over the last couple of decades with a demand that leaders need to be drawn from the ranks of nursing more so than in the past (Cox & le May, 2007). In order to be an effective leader and by implication a practising change-agent in the future, one of the key requirements is to develop a sufficient power base so that one can exercise authority. Handy (1999) identifies four sources of power which can be used either in isolation or collectively, and these are referred to as position, resource, personal and expert or knowledge power. To an extent, the acquisition of expert or knowledge power is derived from one's professional status. However, the nurse must also recognise that professional development is an on-going expectation and responsibility that is assumed by the individual who enjoys the privilege of describing himself or herself as a professional. This is of course explicitly recognised within the NMC Code (2008). Continuous educational development is therefore a hallmark of being a professional and this will feature in the ability of a practitioner to accumulate a sufficient basis of power, in what is one of the most recognisable and legitimate sources (expert/knowledge) of those identified by Handy (1999).

Leadership approaches

In addition to developing a sufficient power base, effective leaders in the future will need to distinguish between what the main theoretical approaches are within contemporary debates about leadership. The two approaches which are used as a means of both contrasting them, whilst offering the prospect that they may also be used in a complementary way are the so-called *transactional* and *transformational* approaches.

Burns (1978) views transactional leadership as being mainly concerned with the exchange of rewards that the leader or manager is able to give in return for specified work. Reciprocity then is a significant element in the relationship between those who lead and the led. Leadership is, therefore, about practically enabling and equipping staff to invest considerable effort. In contrast to this, transformational leadership, which enjoys a good deal of contemporary exposure with such influential organisations as the NHS Leadership and Innovation Unit, is more about leaders helping their staff to willingly transform themselves and the way they are able to perform in the work place. This somewhat puts leadership on a higher plain and as Peters and Waterman (1988) state, it involves leaders and followers engaging in such a way that they can achieve higher levels of motivation and indeed morality. The implication of this is that staff cannot be led any longer in the more traditional command–control approach, but they require a style from their leaders that is much more consistent with their higher educational standing and a requirement for a greater level of involvement in how the work is carried out.

In order to develop the ability to act as a leader, consistent with a more transformational approach, the NHS Leadership Qualities Framework, developed by the NHS Leadership Centre (2002) highlights the challenges faced by health care professionals in leadership roles and these include issues such as the change agenda, service improvement, flexibility, the needs of patients and greater accountability. As a practical means of promoting the behaviour that might become associated with being an effective leader, Stewart (1989) has suggested that the budding leader needs to develop in five key areas (Box 7.3, Activity 7.2).

> **BOX 7.3**
>
> **Five key leadership areas (Stewart 1989)**
>
> - Setting an example
> - Developing your 'image'
> - Projecting self-confidence
> - Influencing others
> - Establishing personal authority.

> **Activity 7.2**
>
> Think of an example under each of these five key areas which might help you in enhancing your standing as a leader?

Developing Your Role in 'Liaison'

A key constant contained with working in health and social care is that it is rare to work in isolation. The white paper *New NHS, Modern, Dependable* (DH 1997) stressed the need for greater cooperation, collaboration and partnership, in replacing the perceived divisiveness associated with a structure within health and social care which appeared to favour competition. Since the white paper there has been a whole plethora of policy-driven reforms which have advocated a more inclusive approach to how health and social care is both structured and delivered. One such initiative, particularly relevant to health and social care professionals who have recently undergone their training, is the emphasis on inter-professional education.

This is reflected in the creation and development, for example, of integrated care pathways, which are now commonly mentioned as an established way by which many patients can be treated concerning a variety of conditions. In order to take advantage of such initiatives, the challenge for all health care professionals is to eradicate the old barriers associated with professional rivalries and to work in a more collaborative and integrated way. Apart from anything else, this should lead to less duplication and ultimately will serve the interests of the patient/client.

This calls for recognition of the important role the individual plays within the multi-disciplinary team and a realisation of the skills and qualities that they are able to bring to it. One useful way of considering the qualities that a team might possess is to reflect on the work of Belbin (1981) and his assertion that in order for a team to be effective it needs to be composed of not necessarily the brightest, but certainly the best. The eight key roles are comprised of chairperson, shaper, plant, monitor-evaluator, resource investigator, company worker, team worker and completer-finisher. Although it might be more natural to consider these roles as those that could make up a management team, they do, however, offer an important insight to the personal qualities within your possession that help you function effectively as a team member. Increasingly, multi-disciplinary teams reach beyond the normal organisational boundaries that we might have identified with in the past and so liaison skills are required at the various interfaces affecting health and social care.

This will include developing relationships with professionals and workers in both acute and community settings, some of whom will be operating in the public, private and voluntary sectors. Liaison then needs to be considered in respect of how an individual is able to develop and maintain relationships not only within the host organisation, most commonly with fellow professionals, but also increasingly in connecting with those in other organisations who will have an important role to play in ensuring care is seamless and consistent. If this is added to the emphasis that there needs to be placed on greater patient and service user involvement, through such agencies as the Patient Advice and Liaison Service (PALS), then developing key management skills in this area becomes an even more pressing necessity.

Informational or Administrating Roles

The roles covered under this heading are broadly concerned with the important functional roles of being an effective 'communicator'. The principles of effective communication are implicit within many of the NMC's (2007) Essential Skills Clusters competency statements within the 'Organisational Aspects of Care' performance criteria, for example, in 'responding to feedback from patients/ clients' and in 'promoting continuity when care is transferred to another service or person'. Communication as a topic is also dealt with in some depth elsewhere in Chapters 1–4 of this book and so the development of these key roles will be addressed relatively briefly here.

Developing your role as a 'monitor', 'disseminator' and 'spokesperson'

Over recent years there has been an exponential rise in the demand for information within the world of health and social care. According to Cooke *et al.* (2004) there is the need to transfer information at all levels and in various ways. They cite the example of the need to exchange information between service users and care staff. In addition, care staff themselves have to provide information for each other by way of such things as care plans and progress of treatment reports. Finally, care staff and their managers need to exchange information regarding such issues as budget reports, performance indicators and new policy initiatives. The ability to be able to process information will therefore be crucial to an individual's success as a manager of care. However, faced with the volume of information that they are often confronted with, part of the skill of a manager of care is in determining what information is useful. In other words, it is about distinguishing valuable information from that which has little or no value.

With this in mind the manager of care needs to *monitor* what information is available and this might involve searching for data from a variety of sources which will be both formal, such as developments in practice and recommendations coming from such bodies as the National Institute for Health and Clinical Excellence

---

BOX 7.4

Communication principles (Wise 2006)

- Communication is a means, not an end
- The context, or situation, affects what needs to be communicated
- The purpose of the communication defines who needs to send a message to whom and provides clues as to how it can best be transmitted
- Feedback needs to be heeded to evaluate communication effectiveness – is the understanding what was intended?
- Collaborating to solve complex problems requires effective communication skills.

Activity 7.3

Identify one thing you could do in order to improve your communication skills in the following areas:
- Talking to patients and members of the public?
- Speaking on the telephone?
- Verbal reporting at 'handover'?
- Written notes?
- Making a formal presentation to colleagues?

(NICE), policy proposals from the Department of Health, and more informally, information that is gleaned from talking to respected colleagues inside and outside of the organisation. Once the information has been deciphered, another key responsibility for managers under this set of roles is to then *disseminate* the relevant information to others in the organisation, who will usually be colleagues.

In this sense the manager of care needs to ensure and encourage the flow of information and to receive feedback from other practitioners as to its usefulness and what are the implications for practice. Having received the responses from other colleagues within the clinical area, the manager is then in a position to fulfil what is identified as the third role within this category, which is to act as a *spokesperson* on behalf of the department or organisation, for example in requesting additional resources necessary to fulfil a new development in practice. In ensuring that one's communication is effective, some important principles have been identified by Yoder Wise (2006) and act as a useful check list or reminder for good managers of care (Box 7.4, Activity 7.3).

Decisional or Fixing Roles

According to Mintzberg (1998), this category of roles is the most important part of managerial activity. It represents the real work in the sense that it involves getting things done and so it is of a very practical nature. From the manager of care's perspective, it also involves the sorts of activities which contribute towards the standing and reputation a manager has. In short, managers should after all be assessed by their ability to be able to get things done.

Developing Your Role as an 'Entrepreneur'

Although the normal dictionary definition of an 'entrepreneur' will refer to someone who undertakes a commercial venture, in most cases, regarding management in a health and social care context, it is more appropriate to think of it in terms of exploiting opportunities. This goes to the heart of the change-management expectation that is an integral part of being seen as a transformational leader. All change should be essentially about improving quality, and over the past 20 years or so, the requirement to focus on patients/clients as consumers, has gathered pace (Carter 2007). This theme of quality dominates the content of Labour's first white paper on health since coming to power in 1997 and in 1998 with the publication of *A First Class Service* (DH 1998), the blueprint for a fully accountable quality assurance framework was outlined in what has become known as 'clinical governance'. In keeping with the principles underpinning 'total quality management (TQM)' (Oakland 1993), there should be the pursuit of continuous quality.

From a management of care point of view this means constantly striving to improve the level of care. This being the case, a key responsibility of all professional nurses should be about adapting and innovating new practice. This needs to be driven by a well-established basis of evidence and should be consistent with the resource limitations (see concepts of *demands, constraints and choices* above) in which the management of care takes place. A manager, therefore, needs to be seen as someone who is able to exploit opportunities for improving practice, and not only does this fulfil a nurse's professional obligation (NMC 2008), but as Handy (1999) states, it also recognises that change is synonymous with the responsibility of management (Activity 7.4).

Activity 7.4

Identify an aspect of nursing practice that requires improvement in the clinical area where you work. How do you intend to take this forward with your colleagues?

Developing Your Role as a 'Disturbance Handler'

In highly complex situations involving the management of care, there are inevitably times when a manager has to deal with unexpected crises and will need to resolve conflicts between staff, professionals and in interactions with patients/clients and their families. Good managers are those who not only can deal with events in such a way that causes the minimum of disruption, but are able to prevent these occurrences happening in the first place. The key to working effectively within this role is to maintain a balance between being able to behave reactively, and at the same time being proactive in minimising the possibility for problems to arise in the first place. If one takes another example from the NMC's Essential Skills Clusters, registered nurses are expected to 'respond appropriately to feedback from patients/clients, the public and a wide range of sources as a vehicle for learning and development' (NMC 2007, p. 12). It goes on to state that this involves nurses responding appropriately to feedback by way of complaints and actively seeking opportunities which should be shared with others in order to learn for future practice. Such an illustration is consistent with the aims of the clinical governance ethos and system which should exist in all health care practice environments.

Good managers of care not only have to be skilled in dealing with situations of conflict as and when they take place, but they also have to plan ahead so that such situations do not arise in the future. Using an approach which has been coined by Parsley and Corrigan (1999) as ensuring 'zero-defects' the aim should be to ultimately eliminate all mistakes that occur, so that eventually no complaints will be necessary. Whilst this may be idealistic in the extreme, it is difficult to contest with what is such a worthy aim, and it remains consistent with the principles of TQM referred to elsewhere in this chapter. Although the handling of complaints is but one example of the manager of care occupying the role of 'disturbance handler' there are, however, some shared elements to how they might practice their management skills which could be common to many other situations involving unscheduled crises. This might involve an approach to one's practice which is underpinned by honesty and ethical principles (Beauchamp & Childress 2001), and guided by objectivity and established procedure. In terms of its execution, one will need to be adept in the techniques of de-escalation and negotiation, and so the ability to display advanced communication skills will be vital. A useful approach to conflict resolution, identified in Box 7.5, has been described by Sullivan and Decker (2005) and involves a number of key rules (Box 7.6).

BOX 7.5

Conflict resolution (Sullivan & Decker 2005)

1. Put the focus on interests by examining and responding to the 'real' issues.
2. Build in opportunities to return to negotiation so that the consequences of failure are fully understood by all and considered unacceptable – this will build commitment.
3. Build in consultation opportunities before and feedback after negotiations – this ensures open discussion and helps to avoid similar conflicts in the future.
4. Provide the necessary motivation, skills and resources – these are key responsibilities of the manager of care who ultimately has to resolve the conflict.

BOX 7.6

Key rules (Sullivan & Decker 2005)

1. Protect each party's self-respect by focusing on issues not personalities.
2. Do not apportion blame but focus on the solution.
3. Encourage open and complete discussion.
4. Allow each party to have equal say regardless of their difference in status.
5. Encourage the full expression of positive and negative feelings.
6. Make sure both parties listen actively.
7. Identify key themes in the discussion and refer to them frequently.
8. Encourage each party to feedback to each other's comments to encourage full understanding.
9. Help the parties to agree and arrive at a mutually acceptable solution.
10. At an agreed interval follow up the progress of the plan.
11. Positively feedback to the participants regarding their cooperation in solving the conflict.

Developing Your Role as a 'Resource Allocator'

Whether the practice setting is located within a public, private or voluntary sector organisation, the challenge of being able to manage and deliver care within limited and finite resources will be something that has to be faced by all managers of care. With the increasing autonomy that nurses have acquired in the way that they practice, the types of resources that have to be considered now go beyond the traditional view of financial, technical/equipment and human resources. Increasingly, professional nurses also have to consider the way that they schedule time in terms of dividing and coordinating the work of others. In the current resource-driven environment in which health care is delivered, nurses need to do more than simply a good job with limited means. They also need to find ever-increasing ways to use such finite resources efficiently (Sullivan & Decker 2005).

One particular approach to the allocation of resources is through the direction and co-ordination of the work of others. *Delegation* is a useful technique for all managers of care to use. It involves the need to bridge what might be described as the dilemma that many reluctant delegators experience, that is the willingness to sacrifice control in order to trust someone else to get on with the delegated task. Delegation then is the process by which responsibility and authority are transferred to another individual (Sullivan & Decker 2005). Accountability remains with the delegator, but the person who takes on the task is also accountable to the delegator for the responsibilities that have been assumed. If delegation is carried out effectively, it can achieve a great deal, for example the manager of care can accomplish more tasks, thereby increasing productivity, and it is also used as a technique to develop skills and abilities within the staff group, and so in this sense it is a very useful and effective developmental device. Marquis and Huston (2006) provide a useful checklist which conforms to the principles of effective delegation (Box 7.7).

BOX 7.7

Principles of effective delegation (Marquis & Huston 2006)

- Plan ahead
- Identify the necessary skills and level required
- Select the most capable person
- Communicate what is to be achieved clearly
- Empower the delegate
- Set deadlines and monitor progress
- Model the role by providing guidance
- Evaluate performance
- Reward accomplishment.

Developing Your Role as a 'Negotiator'

Pugh and Hickson (1996) interpret this final role that Mintzberg (1998) identified as being about the manager needing to negotiate with others and in the process make sound decisions about the commitment of organisational resources. The necessity to exercise good negotiating skills will be determined by a variety of reasons, not least the examples cited above such as conflict resolution or delegation. Successful negotiation, however, represents real achievement for the aims of the organisation, and the interests of the patient/client should be synonymous with this. The manager of care therefore has to negotiate with other managers, members of staff and patients/clients and their families. Once again, this calls for a set of skills which are based on excellent personal communication and organisational abilities. It might involve acting as an advocate in protecting the interests and rights of a patient/client. Similarly, one might have to negotiate for additional resources from those in authority. This could be because of a belief that patient/client care is being compromised and an unacceptable level of risk is present.

Conclusion

Handy (1999, p. 322) states, 'the problem, if it is a problem, is one of roles'. All managers have an array of roles which they need to occupy and the range can seem overwhelming, particularly when one considers the host of skills and knowledge required to operate effectively within them. The challenge of management is so comprehensive and all consuming that some way of attempting to categorise managerial roles should be helpful, which is why the approach taken in this chapter is so. That is not to say that the review of activities present here is by any means comprehensive. In that sense it is consistent with the generally held view that management is a dynamic and eclectic function which calls for the practice of a vast array of skills. The challenges for a professional nurse taking on the mantle of a manager of care are considerable. It is yet another manifestation of the transformation in the identity of the modern-day professional nurse (Activity 7.5).

Activity 7.5

Additional reading and resources

Broome A. (1998) *Managing Change*, 2nd edn. Macmillan, Basingstoke (Essentials of Nursing Management Series).

Finkelman A.W. (2006) *Leadership and Management in Nursing*. Prentice Hall, New Jersey.

Girvin J. (1998) *Leadership and Nursing*, 2nd edn. Macmillan, Basingstoke (Essentials of Nursing Management Series).

Hewison A. (2004) *Management for Nurses and Health Professionals*. Blackwell, Oxford.

Matthews A. (1993) *In Charge of the Ward*, 3rd edn. Blackwell, Oxford.

Tschudin V., Schober J. (1998) *Managing Yourself*, 2nd edn. Macmillan, Basingstoke (Essentials of Nursing Management Series).

Woodhall G., Stuttard A. (1999) *Financial Management*. Macmillan, Basingstoke (Essentials of Nursing Management Series).

Section 2

References

Beauchamp T.L., Childress J.F. (2001) *Principles of Biomedical Ethics*, 5th edn. Oxford University Press, New York.

Belbin R.M. (1981) *Management Team*. Heinemann, Oxford.

Burns J. (1978) *Leadership*. Harper and Row, New York.

Carter R. (2007) Quality and clinical governance (Chapter 8). In: *Principles of Professional Studies in Nursing* (eds Brown J., Libberton P.). Palgrave, Basingstoke.

Cooke S., Henderson E., Martin V., Bak E. (2004) *Managing Information – Module 4 of Managing in Health and Social Care*. Open University, Milton Keynes.

Cox Y., le May A. (2007) Quality and clinical governance (Chapter 9). In: *Principles of Professional Studies in Nursing* (eds Brown J., Libberton P.). Palgrave, Basingstoke.

Department of Health (DH) (1997) *The New NHS: Modern, Dependable*. The Stationery Office, London.

Department of Health (DH) (1998) *A First Class Service*. The Stationery Office, London.

Department of Health (DH) (2000) *The NHS Plan: A Plan for Investment, a Plan for Reform*. The Stationery Office, London.

European Union (1993) *E U Working Time Directive*. Council Directive 93/104/EC. The Council of The European Union, Brussells.

Fayol H. (1949) *General and Industrial Management*. Pitman, London.

The Guardian (2008) Guardian Newspaper, 7th January 2008.

Hales C. (1993) *Managing Through Organisation*. Routledge, London.

Handy C. (1999) *Understanding Organizations*. Penguin, London.

Humphris D., Masterton A. (eds) (2000) *Developing New Clinical Roles: A Guide for Health Professionals*. Churchill Livingstone, Edinburgh.

Hunter D. (2003) *Public Health Policy*. Polity, Oxford.

Marquis B.L., Huston C.J. (2006) *Leadership Roles and Management Functions in Nursing*, 5th edn. Lippincott, Philadelphia.

Mintzberg H. (1998) *Covert Leadership: Notes on Managing Professionals*. Harvard Business Review, November–December, pp.140–147.

Nolan Committee (1996) *First Report on Standards in Public Life*. The Stationery Office, London.

NHS Leadership Centre (2002) *NHS Leadership Qualities Framework*. DH, London.

Nursing and Midwifery Council (NMC) (2007) *Essential Skills Clusters*. NMC Circular 07(2007) Annexe 2, NMC, London.

Nursing and Midwifery Council (NMC) (2008) *The Code: Standards of Conduct, Performance and Ethics for Nurses and Midwives*. Nursing and Midwifery Council, London.

Oakland J. (1993) *Total Quality Management*, 2nd edn. Heinemann, Oxford.

Parsley K., Corrigan P. (1999) *Quality Improvement in Health Care*. Stanley Thornes, Cheltenham.

Peters T.J., Waterman R.H. (1988) *In Search of Excellence*. Harper and Row, New York.

Pugh D.S., Hickson D.J. (1996) *Writers on Organizations*, 5th edn. Penguin, London.

Stewart R. (1982) *Choices for the Manager*. McGraw Hill, Maidenhead.

Stewart R. (1989) *Leading in the NHS: A Practical Guide*. Macmillan, Houndmills.

Sullivan E.J., Decker P.J. (2005) *Effective Leadership and Management in Nursing*, 6th edn. Pearson, New Jersey.

UKCC (1992) *Scope of Professional Practice*. UKCC, London.

Wilkinson J.M. (2007) *Nursing Process and Critical Thinking*. Prentice Hall, London.

Yoder Wise P.S. (2006) *Leading and Managing in Nursing*, 4th edn. Mosby, St Louis.

CHAPTER 8

Promoting Health and Well-being

Wendy Wigley and Lyn Wilson

Introduction

This chapter aims to explore the concept of promoting health and well-being. The first part of the chapter investigates what is meant by a health-promoting approach, discusses the determinants of health, and explores the social, environmental, spiritual and individual issues which impact on health status. The second half considers the relevance of these issues to contemporary nursing practice, particularly in relation to the protection of vulnerable individuals. The chapter also offers a framework for encouraging behaviour change – an important skill for all nurses promoting health and well-being.

The specific learning outcomes addressed in this chapter link with the Nursing and Midwifery Council's (NMC 2007) Essential Skills Clusters, and are identified below.

Learning outcomes

By the end of this chapter you will be able to do the following:

- Recognise what is meant by a health-promoting approach.
- Identify the determinants of health and understand their impact on health and well-being.
- Describe a range of models of 'health'.
- Recognise the role of the nurse in promoting health with vulnerable individuals.
- Appreciate the use of health behaviour change frameworks to guide health-promoting practices.

Promoting Health

Whilst working as a Health Promotion Specialist and a Specialist Community Public Health Nurse (Health Visitor) we became frustrated by the way that health promotion was often (*mis*)described as health *promotions*, implying that it is merely a healthy version of a sales and marketing approach. The much-quoted World Health Organisation (WHO) defines health promotion as 'the process of enabling people to increase control over, and to improve, their health' (WHO 1984, cited in Ewles & Simnett 2003, p. 23); however, this definition does not particularly assist us. Although the definition describes the ultimate *aim* of health promotion activity, there is little reference as to *how* this is to be achieved. Health promotion can sometimes remain a rather mysterious process; something vague happens, which does not involve medicines or treatment, and people 'become' healthier.

The reality is that effective health promotion is a complex, multi-pronged approach to improving the health of an identified population. The process aims for empowerment of individuals, rather than coercion or concordance. The main tasks are; to increase people's knowledge about how and why they should select a healthier route; to give them the skills to undertake the new choice; and to influence attitudes so that individuals, groups and communities become more willing and able to make healthier choices.

Planning and provision of health promotion activities is therefore fraught with difficult decisions, some of which are outlined below:

1. *Who* are the identified population?
2. *Why* should we target them?
3. *How* can we influence knowledge, skills and attitudes?
4. *Should we* be influencing knowledge, skills and attitudes?
5. What is our *evidence* that the approach is ethical?
6. Will we get value for money?
7. *How* will we know whether the activity has 'worked'?

And once the activity is under way, we should consider the following on an ongoing basis:

8. Are we *involving* the appropriate people in an effective way?
9. Have we got the *outcome* we expected?
10. Should we *change* what we are doing?

See Activity 8.1.

Activity 8.1

Are these questions, 1–10 above, only pertinent to the practice of health promotion? Which of these questions would be applicable to nursing practice and when?

Think about the nursing process, the process has four main components: *assessment, planning, implementation and evaluation.* Decide which of the above questions apply to which nursing process component. For example, asking 'Who should we involve?' is part of the *assessment* process.

Although the process of promoting health may seem daunting, some of the considerations are not that different from the sometimes difficult decisions made and skills implemented in day-to-day nursing practice.

What is a 'Health-promoting' Approach?

A useful starting point for answering this question is the consideration of different perspectives on the meaning of 'health'. The idea of health being more than 'not being ill' is a long-standing one; the 1946 constitution of the WHO described health as 'a state of complete physical, mental and social well-being and not merely the absence of disease or infirmity' (WHO 1946, p. 2).

Broadly speaking, four perspectives on health can be identified and these are listed as follows:

- The medical model of health
- The holistic model or 'holism'
- The social model of health
- The salutogenic model.

We have to keep in mind that health promotion approaches aim to *empower* individuals, groups and communities; that is, to improve their *own* health through their *own* actions. Below we describe these four models and explore the relevance of each model from a health-promoting perspective.

The medical model of health

The *medical* model defines health as an absence of disease. This understanding of health has historically been the prevailing account in the Western medical profession and the approach can be described as 'medicalisation' (Black & Gruen 2005). The medical model considers that medical influence and control are beneficial for health. However, the model has major limitations, particularly when applied to health promotion.

The premise of the medical approach is that disease can be reduced through treatment and that the application of treatment requires expert knowledge and intervention. A medical approach in public health requires the identification of illness and disease risk factors, with a subsequent focus on identification of those at risk via screening programmes and treatment interventions. This model is criticised for its focus on illness, the assumption that treatment will cure illness and the conclusion that ill health is often caused by individuals 'doing' the wrong thing (Black & Gruen 2005; Lucas & Lloyd 2005). Public health workers, professionals working in social care and the public can perceive the approach as victim blaming and disempowering. The medical model may fail to recognise, for example, that a person with disabilities or a long-term condition can live a healthy life, albeit within the context and constraints of their condition or disability (Davidson 2005; Department of Health (DH) 2006).

The medical model approach, in its most extreme version, focuses only on how a body functions and simply treats the disability or illness rather than enabling the person to live to the best of his or her capabilities. We believe therefore that this model is insufficient for a health-promoting approach. Medical treatment and interventions may be required to 'restore' health, but the skill of promoting health is to enable individuals to become *empowered* so as to improve their own health through knowledge and skills. Ensuring that structures, systems and provision in our society are designed to improve health is an important aspect of health promotion not encompassed by the medical approach.

The holistic model

Black and Gruen (2005) define *holism* as viewing the patient or client 'as a whole (with) the belief that the whole is greater than the sum of the parts' (Black & Gruen 2005, p. 235). The *holistic* model of health is common to the approach preferred by nurses, health professionals, complementary therapists and social care professionals. When assessing the health of an individual, mental health, biological aspects and social aspects are taken into account; that is, mind, body and soul are considered. The idealistic practicalities of this approach have been widely debated (Porter 1997). For example, if an individual is admitted to hospital with asthma, the asthma would be treated and the person sent home. However, a full holistic assessment might reveal that the individual lived in damp accommodation that was affected by damp and mildew, which is known to have a detrimental affect on asthma (Sandel & Wright 2006). In this example, better-quality housing might be the factor that would be most likely to improve health, but this factor would be seen to be outside the remit of the National Health Services (NHS). The NHS focus is likely to be on individual treatment, care and rehabilitation.

The holistic model is limited then in its applicability to health promotion, as there can be a focus on dealing with individuals rather than groups or communities. In addition, Porter (1997) debates the realities of a 'holistic' approach for those health and social care workers whose professional role involves 'surveillance' of a particular client group. The example above demonstrates the limitations of a 'holistic' approach. While the nurse undertaking an assessment might realise that what the individual really requires to improve his or her health is better housing, to access new housing the individual would have to attend a housing service and be reassessed. The philosopher Foucault (1973) criticised the holistic approach as being 'the gaze of the state'. He argued that surveillance increases tension and anxiety, as people can feel guilty when their lifestyles are questioned and criticised. The implications of surveillance and subsequent feelings of guilt are inappropriate to an empowering approach (Earle 2007a).

Despite this debate the practice of holism as a model for nursing practice is a positive concept and an essential nursing skill. Nursing practice should view the individual as a total system, recognising that health is influenced by internal and external environments and acknowledging the uniqueness of individual life.

The social model of health

Encompassed in the *social* model is the idea (or concept) that health is influenced by political, economic, social, psychological, cultural, environmental and biological factors. Proponents of this model argue that concepts of health are socially constructed and therefore we need to understand the subjective (i.e. individual) experience of health, illness and disease (Earle 2007a). The social model of health is very appropriate to health-promotion practice, particularly as the approach advocates *involvement, empowerment* and *partnership* as the main means of improving health and reducing inequalities. Current government policy initiatives are purported to be based on a 'social model', but the reality of achieving this approach has been critiqued. Many government policies reflect a medical approach with an emphasis on factors and circumstances that impede the health of individuals' health – rather than those that promote good health within communities (Hunter 2007). As a consequence the targets set continue to focus on he measurement of disease or treatment incidence. For example, the new ten-year Drug Strategy, *Drugs: Protecting Families and Communities* (Home Office 2008), requires Drug and Alcohol Action Teams to work to increase the number of clients in treatment, bring about reductions in drug-related crime rates and increase the number of individuals offered treatment regimes rather than prison sentences. Despite a new focus in this strategy of working with families, these targets could continue to encourage a 'harm minimisation' approach, with a tokenistic consideration of the reasons why people misuse substances.

Government policy since 1997 has considered wider community benefits, for example, in area-based regeneration initiatives such as New Deal or Sure Start. However, these initiatives are often subject to individual and separate funding streams which restrict service providers' abilities to implement and manage new initiatives cohesively alongside other service provision (Hunter 2007). As a result, such initiatives are sometimes criticised as prompting a so-called post code lottery. For example, Sure Start initiatives have made resources available to the most socially deprived areas but families and children living just outside these areas can be denied access (Earle 2007b). Despite intent to pursue a social model of health, financial and spending restraints can lead to a targeted, risk-identifying and, ultimately, a medical model approach to improving health.

The salutogenic model

Aaron Antonovsky was the main proponent of the *salutogenic* concept of health, which focuses on what keeps people healthy rather than what makes people ill (Antonovsky 1979). He argued that illness, stress and disruption are an unavoidable and normal part of life. Although homeostatic (i.e. balancing) mechanisms within an individual attempt to maintain health, Antonovsky asserted that existence within a continuum from disease to health is a more realistic expectation than continual good health. With these beliefs in mind, Antonovsky coined the phrase *salutogenesis*, explaining that the human condition is to produce health and combat disease through a positive process. Through research over many years, Antonovsky (1996) attempted to uncover successful coping mechanisms: what he called *salutary* factors. He examined concentration camp survivors, trying to find out what had helped them to cope with the extreme adverse conditions. He named his main construct 'sense of coherence' (SOC), arguing that people with a strong SOC would cope better in difficult situations. He also suggested that SOC had three components; if a situation was perceived as *comprehensible, manageable* and *meaningful,* a person would find it easier to cope with the situation. Antonovsky and his work has proved to be a powerful advocate for health-promoting activities which strengthen an individual's capacity to cope; that is, activities that make life more comprehensible, manageable and meaningful for an individual, a group or a community (Antonovsky 1996).

Like Antonovsky, health promoters prefer to take a positive approach to maintenance of health. The philosophy of empowerment is that people are encouraged to discover what helps to keep *them* healthy and therefore Antonovsky's ideas are pertinent to a health-promoting approach. Antonovsky's work has been criticised for focusing on individuals and failing to recognise the impact of wider social factors on health. However, Antonovsky (1996) argues that identification of factors impacting on an individual's health should lead to structural, political and economic changes to support positive health; the onus for change is not just on the individual.

Lay Accounts of Health

Researchers have found that lay people draw on a rich variety of experiences and insights in order to make sense of what health means to them. Shaw (2002) argues that lay understandings are often informed (or *mis*informed) to some extent by an 'expert', such as a general practitioner (GP), a nurse, a book or the internet. Within nursing practice, lay knowledge should be handled sensitively and respected. Figure 8.1 demonstrates that most care provision is provided from and within the home bringing the nurse into contact with a range of family members, carers and other supporters. Clients, families and their carers often hold a 'body of knowledge'

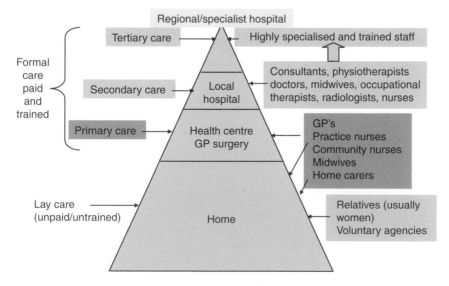

Figure 8.1　Formal and lay care patterns of provision (Wigley 2008).

about health and illness that are integral to their culture, even providing the basis to the beliefs and values of the culture. Skinner (1971) would describe these ideas and values as 'social contingencies' (Skinner 1971, p. 126) arguing that the exposure of an individual to these ideas and values enables the culture to be 'self-perpetuating' (Skinner 1971, p. 127). This means that beliefs about health and disease can be intransigent (i.e. difficult to change).

Many of you may have heard from older relatives, say grandparents, that sitting on cold damp ground can lead to piles (medically known as haemorrhoids), that rubbing goose fat on your chest helps cure a cold and that if you have a burn or a bump you should rub butter on it. Of course, there is no evidence to suggest that any of these are based on fact, but they are an example of knowledge and beliefs handed down through generations. Professionals know such 'old wives tales' to be myths, but nurses should remember that professional scientific knowledge should not be used as 'power' over and above lay knowledge. One should not consider lay knowledge as 'wrong' but as 'different'. A nurse's attempt to dismiss lay knowledge can impact upon the clients self-belief, may stigmatise and 'pigeon hole' the client and, additionally, can remove from the client values and beliefs held as a form of self-protection. For example, when discussing the benefits of stopping smoking with clients we have often heard expressions such as 'My grandmother smoked all her life and lived to be ninety two!' Grandma may well have done, and it is not the role of the nurse to dispute this.

Ideological definitions and understandings of health within the establishment, society, communities, groups or individuals will influence the extent to which any health promotion activity is successful as these understandings will influence the planning (what is to be done?), delivery (how is it to be done?) and evaluation (did the activity achieve what it set out to achieve?). Partnership working between client, patient or carer is very important in health-promotion practice, but it is not easy. One of the reasons for this, as we have demonstrated above, is that different partners often hold differing ideological approaches and understandings of health, making it difficult to agree on decisions, influence change, or identify a way forward. As Ewles and Simnett (2003) suggest, professional knowledge can often embody government ideology and therefore, as nurses, we must guard against promoting social manipulation which represents the views of a prevailing social class but may be to the disadvantage of others in the population.

What Determines Health Status?

Within the field of public health there is a clear recognition that health is determined not just by absence of disease but by many factors, including individual characteristics, society, culture and the environment. The acknowledgement of the many causes of poor health, illness, disease and premature death was neatly summarised in a model devised by Dahlgren and Whitehead (2007) (Figure 8.2).

The model was originally known as 'the policy rainbow', as the authors wished to impress on policy makers the impact of policy decisions on health. Certainly in the United Kingdom, throughout the 1970s and 1980s, the political influence and emphasis for health and health promotion was on lifestyle factors and the

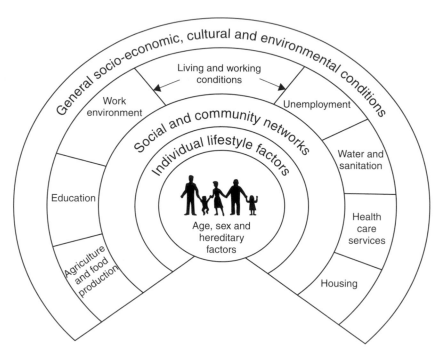

Figure 8.2   Health and influences on levels of health (determinants of health, Dahlgren & Whitehead 2007). Reproduced with the kind permission of Institute of Future Studies, Sweden. (Dahlgren G., Whitehead M. (1992) *Policies and Strategies to Promote Social Equity in Health.* WHO, Copenhagen.)

role of the individuals in improving their own health (Pearson 2003). There was little recognition of the potential contribution of government action to improve health.

At the centre of Dahlgren and Whitehead's model are fixed individual characteristics including age, sex and genetic make up. The next layer of influence is lifestyle factors such as whether a person smokes, the food he or she eats, the amount of exercise he or she takes and the risky behaviours that he or she may or may not indulge in. The third ring could be described as immediate environmental factors. It includes obvious environmental factors such as condition of housing, sanitation and access to recreational space, but also determinants such as whether a person has a job, his or her social networks and support systems. The outer ring also describes environmental and cultural factors, but from a national, rather than local, perspective. This ring therefore includes government policies to protect or maintain health; the provision of universal services such as education and health services, agriculture and food provision; and the standard of living conditions – pollution, rates of employment and health and safety at work.

The Dahlgren and Whitehead model has been much used by researchers as a framework for exploring the size of the contribution of different determinants. In the past the causes of poor health, illness, disease and early death have sometimes been identified as the outcome of individual lifestyle choice. However, evidence demonstrates that, although some social groups have much higher rates of illness,

---

Activity 8.2

Question: Look again at Figure 8.2; can you identify *how* the determinants of health might impact upon an individual, group or community? Here are some ideas we have considered:

- The quality and suitability of housing may be influenced by employment status.
- Employment status is affected by education and access to transport.
- Loneliness, social isolation and fear of crime are affected by the design and quality of the built environment, mobility and income.
- Income, education and social networks are linked to levels of exercise, adequacy of diet and vulnerability to substance abuse.

---

disease and death than others, these differences cannot be explained solely as a result of adverse lifestyle decisions (Wilkinson *et al.* 1998) (Activity 8.2).

As we discussed earlier, many of these determinants of health lie beyond the reach of health service providers, in the social and economic fabric of society. Improving the health of a society depends on reducing the health inequalities arising from these socio-economic determinants. This means working in partnership with agencies responsible for making decisions about housing, business, transport, leisure, education, and so on, to influence health directly. The important conclusion is that health is determined by many interacting factors, some of which are more important at certain times in a person's life, some of which are under individual control, but many of which are not.

Psychosocial Determinants of Health

Psychosocial determinants are those social factors which impact on the psychology of an individual. From a nursing perspective these determinants are important for several reasons:

- A nurse is more likely to promote health with individuals rather than large groups.
- A nurse may be unable to directly influence economic or structural factors which could improve health.
- A nurse can build a professional relationship with an individual. Nurses can encourage an individual and explain strategies that enable the person to cope more successfully with difficult situations.

There is good evidence to illustrate how a health professional can influence an individual's cognitions (a person's understanding and knowledge of their self and life) (NICE guidance, NICE 2007). Marmot and Wilkinson (2006) have written extensively about how social and economic structures impact on health and they have suggested that psychosocial factors play a large part in determining health status. Marmot and Wilkinson (2006) suggest that there are three main aspects to psychosocial risk factors: *social status*, *social affiliations* and *stress in early life*.

All three aspects are affected by material living standards (i.e. how much money a person has); Marmot and Wilkinson argue that poverty or wealth mediates and defines social position.

Poverty and deprivation

Wigley (2008) argues that poverty is a difficult concept to define in the twenty-first century Western society but suggests poverty is a 'relative' concept, reflecting not only expected human needs but also the requirements, merchandise and life chances available and accepted as 'the norm' by the general public. Many people deemed to be living 'in poverty' may also live in areas of deprivation. The term deprivation is used to describe the ecological aspects of a given area, that is, aspects such as level of income, housing standards, rates of employment, educational qualifications and rates of chronic disease and stress. These aspects are measured using *indices* or *scales*. In 2004, the Indices of Deprivation (ID2004) (Neighbourhood Renewal Unit 2003) were published. These indices are based on 2001 census information and statistical data from governmental departments and take into consideration a variety of indicators, domains and issues, including those listed in Table 8.1.

The deprivation indices were not based upon the previous geographic community and electoral wards as previous statistical indices had been; these were based upon a new geographical conceptual hierarchy known as Super Output Areas (SOAs) (Office for National Statistics 2008) (Activity 8.3).

Table 8.1 Indicators and issues considered in ID2004. *Source*: Neighbourhood Renewal Unit (2003).

Indicators	Issues considered
Income	• Adults and children in Income Support households • Adults and children in Income-based Job Seekers Allowance households • Adults and children in Working Families Tax Credit households (excluding housing benefits) • Adults and children in Disabled Person's Tax Credit households (excluding housing benefits) • Adults and children in households in receipt of National Asylum Support Service (NASS) vouchers
Employment	• Unemployment claimant count (Joint Unemployment & Vacancies Operating System Cohort (JUVOS)) of women aged 18–59 and men aged 18–64 averaged over 4 quarters • Incapacity Benefit claimants women aged 18–59 and men aged 18–64 • Severe Disablement Allowance claimants women aged 18–59 and men aged 18–64 • Participants in New Deal for the 18–24s who are not included in the claimant count • Participants in New Deal for 25+ who are not included in the claimant count • Participants in New Deal for Lone Parents aged 18 and over

(Continued)

Table 8.1 Continued.

Indicators	Issues considered
Health and disability	• Years of Potential Life Lost Comparative Illness and Disability Ratio (CIDR) • Measures of acute • Proportion of the population suffering mental ill health based on prescribing and/or hospital episode
Education, skills and training	• Average points score of children at Key Stage 2 (end of primary) • Average points score of children at Key Stage 3 • Average points score of children at Key Stage 4 (GCSE/GNVQ – best of eight results) • Proportion of young people *not* staying on in school or school level education above 16 • Proportion of those aged under 20 not entering Higher Education • Secondary school absence rate Proportions of working age adults (aged 25–59) in the area with no qualifications
Barriers to housing and services	• Modelled ratio of pre-school children to pre-school child care places • Ratio of GPs per head of population • Household overcrowding (2001, ONS Census) • District level rate of applications under the homelessness provisions of the 1996 Housing Act, assigned to the constituent Super Output Areas (SOAs) • Difficulty of Access to owner-occupation • Road distance to a GP surgery • Road distance to a general stores or supermarket • Road distance to a primary school • Road distance to a Post Office
Crime and disorder	• Offenders • Home contents insurance premiums • Fire data • Fear of crime
Living environment	• Overcrowding • Affordability of housing • Homelessness • Households lacking basic amenities • Children in unsuitable accommodation • Vacant dwellings and low demand • Land use and derelict land

Section 2

Activity 8.3

Go to Neighbourhood Statistics (2008) home page at http://neighbourhood.statistics.gov.uk/dissemination/LeadPage.do?pageId=1001&tc=1205772919507&a=3&i=1001&m=0&s=1205772919507&enc=1

The box on the right-hand side enables you to find a summary report for a local neighbourhood, community or area in which you live or work

Do the statistics you find reflect what you thought or knew about the area?

Were there any statistics that surprised you?

Now complete the box on the left-hand side of the web page, this will give you numerous statistics for your local authority, electoral ward and the name of the SOA.

One of the problems with indices and scales of deprivation (as you may have found) is that terms such as '*poverty*' and '*deprivation*' can be demeaning and reflect an often historical stigma relating to a community and the group or individual who lives within that community (Wigley 2008). An important task for health promoters is to encourage social networks and community action to reduce stigma.

Social status

Social status is thought to influence health through its impact on a persons' sense of personal control; a range of research supports this view. Wilkinson *et al.* (1998) used US data to examine the relationships between various categories of income inequality, state income, social trust and mortality. Their study explored the *social processes* which might account for the relationship between greater income equality and lower population mortality rates. The findings demonstrated that murder rates had an even closer relationship to income inequality than did mortality from all other causes combined. Wilkinson *et al.*'s (1998) data suggest that violent crime is closely related to income inequality, social trust and mortality rates, and feeling shamed, humiliated and disrespected relate to the way in which wider income differences mean more people are denied the traditional sources of status and respect associated with wealth and income. The emotional aspects of low social status may be central to the psychosocial processes linking inequality, violence, social cohesion and mortality (Wilkinson *et al.* 1998).

Work and sickness

The Whitehall study of civil servants (North *et al.* 1996) sought to examine the association between the psychosocial work environment and subsequent rates of sickness absence and found that health worsened the lower down the hierarchy the worker was. Workers at the bottom of the hierarchy were also found to have the least control over their role and workload.

Education and social affiliations

Educational studies (Ross & Broh 2000) have shown that children who perceive a low sense of control over what happens to them at school do least well in exams. Other evidence (Health Development Agency (HDA) 2004) suggests that irregular school attendance and low educational achievement increases the risk of a range of health outcomes for young people including involvement in risky behaviours.

Social affiliations are the practical and emotional supports which can be provided by others close to the individual (Ewles & Simnett 2003). Support is seen as important for building resilience, and someone who is resilient is more able to cope with stressful situations and therefore less likely to experience ill health as a result of stress. The implication for health promotion is that building of social affiliations, also known as *social capital*, should be an important aim. Furthermore, the act of participating, that is, taking a role in decision-making opportunities, has been shown to impact on an individual's sense of personal control (HDA 2004). A health promoter will therefore aim to encourage involvement of communities in the decision-making processes. Not only will the decisions be more relevant to the community but the very act of involvement will strengthen an individual's sense of personal control.

Life course events

Psychosocial circumstances can affect an individual's life course; events in early life can impact on outcomes in later life. Wilkinson (2005) suggests that low birth weight is due to stress during pregnancy rather than a lack of food. Low birth weight individuals have been found to have a higher risk of disease in later life (Barker & Godfrey 2001). Stress and a lack of stimulation in early childhood can also compromise future health and social mobility. Olds *et al.* (1999) undertook a 15-year follow-up of a randomised controlled trial that considered the impact of a programme of prenatal and early childhood home visitation by nurses. The trial demonstrated that home visitation, by nurses in particular, can reduce reported serious antisocial behaviour and substance misuse in adolescents born into high-risk families. The findings of this study resulted last year in the joint Department of Health and Department for Children, Schools and Families pilot of a model of intensive nurse-led home visiting for vulnerable first-time parents. The model is being tested in ten areas in England and involves family nurses visiting young, disadvantaged parents from early pregnancy until the child is 2 years old. Nurses build close, supportive relationships with families and guide inexperienced teenagers to adopt healthier lifestyles, improve their parenting skills and become self-sufficient (Billingham 2007).

Societal equality

Marmot and Wilkinson (2006), somewhat controversially, suggest that egalitarian (i.e. equal or fair) societies tend to have higher standards of health and longevity. What this could mean is that provision of services is not as important as equality in a society. This is challenging to policy makers as it is more difficult to bring about equality than simply improve services. Also, Wilkinson would argue that improving services can sometimes worsen equality, particularly if the services are least accessible to those who are most in need of them. Reducing health inequalities is therefore an important aim of the twenty-first-century health promotion, and there are two main reasons for this. The first is the ethical imperative to ensure equity; those in low socio-economic groups should not have their health compromised by their social position. The second imperative is the reality of limited resources. If resources are limited then the most effective and efficient action is to target those resources to areas in most need. In order to reduce health inequalities health-promotion activity is targeted at areas of deprivation.

Promoting Health and Well-being and Nursing

As nursing adapts to meet the health and social needs of the twenty-first century, there must be an even greater emphasis on prevention of ill health, health promotion and supporting self-care. The DH consultation document, *Towards a Framework for Post-registration Nursing Careers: A National Consultation* (DH 2007), discussed several factors in the case for changing the

Section 2

career structure of nursing practice and expertise and two factors are particularly salient to this discussion:

> Health care must respond to the global shift in the burden of disease that is seeing a rise in the numbers of people affected by one or more long term condition. Many experience both physical and mental health problems at the same time.

> Health inequalities persist despite all efforts to reduce the gap. As well as the disadvantaged, many of those whose physical health is poorest have long term and enduring mental health problems or learning difficulties. (DH 2006, p. 7)

It is the role of the nurse to promote and protect the health and well-being of vulnerable clients or patients (NMC 2007, 2008). Two government documents: *No Secrets: Guidance on Developing and Implementing Multi-agency Policies and Procedures to Protect Vulnerable Adults from Abuse* (DH & Home office 2000) and *Working Together to Safeguard Children* (HM Government 2006) make it clear that the responsibility of protecting vulnerable individuals does not fall to one agency alone. However, it is often the nurse who may be the 'first contact' with vulnerable individuals and their carers, and the principles of effective assessment should remain the same regardless of whether these individuals are adults or children:

- To gather information and recognise the sources of vulnerability.
- To identify strengths and protective factors.
- To identify needs and inconsistencies that influence outcomes.
- To inform action.

The final point may necessitate an immediate discussion with a responsible colleague or another agency, the main priority being to ensure safety and protection. All agencies (statutory and voluntary) and professionals involved with vulnerable individuals and their carers are required to share information when risk and/or abuse is identified, and this commitment overrules any duty of confidentiality (*Public Interest Disclosure Act*, Office of Public Sector Information 1998; Beckett 2005; NMC 2008).

So how can the nurse promote health and well-being?

For health promotion to be effective it is clear that the full range of health determinants must be tackled. The different determinants, such as societal, political, economic and biological, cannot be tackled using one method. The promotion of health and well-being therefore draws on a range of methods, some of which are summarised in Table 8.2. Evidence for what works in health promotion indicates that there should be a concerted effort to address all the determinants of health.

There is good evidence to suggest that nurses should be encouraging individual health-related behaviour change (NICE 2007; NMC 2007). The next section describes a framework for encouraging health behaviour change.

Health Behaviour Change Framework

The health behaviour change framework (Table 8.3) describes the tasks for the health professional when meeting with a patient to discuss health behaviour

Table 8.2   Promotion of health and well-being matrix.

Method	Useful for	Limitations
Health education e.g. teaching skills, increasing knowledge, challenging attitudes.	One-to-one work or small group work where the aim is to influence knowledge, attitudes and skills.	Health education alone is unlikely to have an impact on structural or economic reasons for poor health.
Social marketing e.g. media campaign to encourage stop smoking.	Reaching a widely distributed but particular audience. Improves health behaviour knowledge and access to services.	Support services (e.g. quit groups and nicotine replacement therapy) must already be in place.
Prevention/reduction activities e.g. breast screening, immunisation. Child protection procedures.	Preventing population-wide ill health and/or harm.	False positives in screening Subject to media controversy limiting uptake i.e. Pertussis immunisation in the 1970s and MMR in the 1990s. Risk of being adversarial and/or paternalistic in implementation.
Area-based initiatives e.g. Sure Start, Children's Centres, community development projects.	Working with and for communities to improve their health. Provides the opportunity to tackle a wide range of issues important to the community.	Tokenistic approaches, e.g. where service and provision is already decided but communities are 'consulted' to gain their approval.
Regulatory activities e.g. raising age of sale of cigarettes, establishing smoke-free public places.	Good approach for certain factors as the measures can improve everyone's health in a fair and equitable way.	Government can be reluctant to introduce what are seen as 'nanny state' interventions.
Economic activities e.g. raising taxes on unhealthy products.	Decreases desirability for unhealthy product.	These activities are strongly resisted by commercial institutions as their profits are affected. Can increase health inequalities if the product is more likely to be purchased by the less well off.
Influencing policies e.g. introducing a local breast feeding policy, lobbying for smoke-free places, better public transport, improved food labelling.	Effective policies can bring about changes in conditions of living.	Certain groups may lobby against the policy change, for example those who stand to lose profit because of the changes.
Multi agency partnerships e.g. Local Area Agreements, Local Strategic partnerships.	Brings a range of agencies together to identify and tackle local health needs.	Requires input of resources, trust and commitment to tackle identified needs.

Table 8.3   Health behaviour change framework.

Key Task	What to do
Establish the relationship	The tasks at this stage will vary according to whether this is the first meeting, a subsequent meeting or the last meeting. At a first meeting it is important to help the client to feel at ease, to encourage them to talk and to set the parameters for the meeting. At subsequent meetings you will be reviewing their action plan so an early task would be to praise their achievements, however small. If this is to be their last meeting with you, you need to alert them to the imminent ending of the relationship.
Negotiate the agenda	Check with the client that they are clear that the agenda is to talk about a health-related behaviour change which they wish to make. Reiterate that it is not a 'counselling session' or 'just a chat'; the expectation is that you will help them to identify changes that they wish to make. Encourage the client to be specific and positive about the particular health behaviour change. An expectation of 'wanting to be healthy' is far too vague. 'I want to be a size 12' is also vague, negative and possibly, unrealistic. One of the 'best' ways to fail to make a change is by setting an unrealistic target at the outset. A target to 'eat more healthily' is a much better start, it is positive, and small, specific actions can be identified at the action-planning stage. The wording of targets is important as it can impact on motivation. A target to, 'become a non-smoker' is an achievable aspiration, positive and specific.
Assess the importance of and the confidence in making the particular change	For example ask 'how important is it to you to become a non-smoker?' and 'how confident are you about becoming a non-smoker?' These simple questions will provide you (and the client) with huge insight into whether they wish to change and the reasons why they might not change. You can ask the client to score their feelings using a scale of 1–10, where 1 = low, 10 = high.
Explore importance	You can now use the numerical score to find out more about how important making this change is to them. If the importance is low you could ask, 'what would have to happen for it to become more important for you to make this change?' If importance is low there may be limits to what you can achieve. It may be that the client will not change until there is a crisis or something else in their life changes. Give the client information if they request it. One technique you could try is to encourage the client to look at the benefits and barriers for change; this may tip the balance towards change. If importance is high, then acknowledge this and explain that any relapses may engender feelings of guilt.

(Continued)

Table 8.3   Continued.

Key Task	What to do
Build confidence	Now discuss the score for confidence. Confidence can vary in different situations, so ask the client to describe situations when they would not feel confident about making or maintaining a change as this could help them to avoid relapse. If the client is fearful of relapse try 'let's talk through how you could deal with that situation'. Ask them to consider what has worked in the past. Resist the temptation to suggest a string of actions that they could undertake; as soon as you state 'you should …' you will encounter resistance. One method that does work is to say 'in my experience I have found that other people in your situation have tried (list ideas) what do you think?' Just changing the wording slightly ensures the emphasis is on possible options which the client could try, rather than it being a list of things they should do. Another useful technique is known as 'a look over the fence'; ask the client to describe 'what it would be like tomorrow if you made this change tonight.'
Negotiate an action plan	Encourage the client to write down actions they will take before the next meeting. Make sure the actions are specific and realistic; e.g. 'eat more fruit'; measurable, e.g. 'eat one piece of fruit'; and time limited, e.g. 'eat one piece of fruit each day'.
Discuss the next steps	Tasks here may include setting a date for the next meeting or saying goodbye.
	Two tasks are ongoing throughout the meeting
Exchanging information	Provide information on the client's terms. Try asking 'what do you need to know about …?' or 'what do you already know about …?' or 'what do you think about what I have told you today?' Again resist the temptation to give information that you think they should have, check out their understanding as the meeting progresses.
Reduce resistance	The aim throughout the meeting is to avoid the client using 'yes, but(s) ….' Your approach is important here, you can make your point of view clear but you must not argue with the client. For example 'I think that (making the change) would improve your health but I hear that you do not want to, is that right?' Instead of arguing try to 'stand alongside' the client and begin to appreciate their point of view. For example, 'what I'm hearing is that it seems unfair to you that others can (state behaviour) for many years and not experience any ill health. How does that make you feel?'

change. The framework relies on the assumption that there are at least ten minutes available for one-to-one discussion and that the patient or client has initiated the conversation. Preferably, there should be opportunities for follow-up discussions, as it is important that the patient can be supported through the process of making a change over time. The framework is based on a model developed by Rollnick *et al.* (1999) and personal experience of training a range of professionals in the use of this model has been drawn upon. The tasks can be useful in encouraging successful behaviour change, although, as Rollnick *et al.* recommend, the framework should not be slavishly adhered to; the health professional needs to develop considerable skill and knowledge to use the framework in a flexible, client-centred way. The Health Trainer manual draws on Rollnick *et al.*'s model and other behaviour change theories and provides some useful tools (Michie *et al.* 2007).

Conclusion

This chapter has discussed the theoretical basis for a health-promoting approach, arguing that if health and keeping well is to be seen as a positive process, then we must understand the role of the many determinants which impact on health status. Health promoters see their role as one of empowerment, enabling individuals, groups or communities to act to improve their own health, on their own terms. We have acknowledged the importance of working in partnership to address social and economic determinants of health; tackling these wider determinants of health is not something that nurses, or any other professional, can achieve alone. We have emphasised the important role of the nurse in promoting health with vulnerable people and in encouraging health behaviour change with those clients or patients who have expressed an interest in making a change.

References

Antonovsky A. (1979) *Health, Stress, and Coping.* Jossey-Bass Inc, San Francisco.

Antonovsky A. (1996) The salutogenic model as a theory to guide health promotion. *Health Promotion International* 11(1): 11–18.

Barker D., Godfrey K. (2001) Fetal nutrition and cardiovascular disease in adult life. In: *Nutritional Health: Strategies for Disease Prevention* (ed. Wilson T., Temple N.). Humana, New Jersey.

Beckett C. (2005) *Child Protection: An Introduction.* Sage, London.

Billingham K. (2007) *DH/DCSF Health-led Parenting Project: Learning from the Family Nurse Partnership Programme.* Department of Health Publications, London, available at http://www.dh.gov.uk

Black N., Gruen R. (2005) *Understanding Health Services.* Open University Press and McGraw Hill Education, Maidenhead.

Dahlgren G., Whitehead M. (2007) *Policies and Strategies to Promote Social Equity in Health.* Background document to WHO – *Strategy Paper for Europe.* Stockholm Institute for Future Studies, Stockholm, Arbetsrapport/Institutet för Framtidsstudier; 2007: 14, available at http://www.framtidsstudier.se/filebank/files/20080109$110739$fil$mZ8UVQv2wQFShMRF 6cuT.pdf (accessed 27 June 2008).

Davidson L. (2005) Recovery, self management and the expert patient – changing the culture of mental health from a UK perspective. *Journal of Mental Health* 14(1): 25–35.

Department of Health (DH) (2006) *Supporting People with Long Term Conditions to Self Care: A Guide to Developing Local Strategies and Good Practice*. Department of Health, London, available at http://www.dh.gov.uk

Department of Health (DH) (2007) *Towards a Framework for Post-registration Nursing Careers – Consultation Document*. Department of Health, London, available at http://www. dh.gov.uk

Department of Health and Home Office (2000) *No secrets: Guidance on Developing and Implementing Multi-agency Policies and Procedures to Protect Vulnerable Adults from Abuse*. DH, London.

Earle S. (2007a) Promoting public health: exploring the issues. In: *Theory and Research in Promoting Public Health* (eds Earle S., Lloyd C., Sidell M., Spurr S.). Sage and The Open University, London, pp. 37–66.

Earle S. (2007b) Focusing on the health of children and young people. In: *Theory and Research in Promoting Public Health* (eds Earle S., Lloyd C., Sidell M., Spurr S.). Sage and The Open University, London, pp. 163–193.

Ewles L., Simnett I. (2003) *Promoting Health: A Practical Guide*. Baillière Tindall, Edinburgh.

Foucault M. (1973) *The Birth of the Clinic: An Archaeology of Medical Perception*. Tavistock, London.

Health Development Agency (HDA) (2004) *Promoting Children and Young People's Participation through the National Healthy School Standard*. Health Development Agency, London.

Home Office (2008) *Drugs: Protecting Families and Communities 2008–2018 Strategy*. The Home Office, London, available at: http://homeoffice.gov.uk

HM Government (2006) *Working Together to Safeguard Children: A Guide to Interagency Working to Safeguard and Promote the Welfare of Children*. The Stationery Office, London.

Hunter D. (2007) Public health policy. In: *Public Health for the 21st Century*, 2nd edn., (eds Orme J., Powell J., Grey M.). Open University Press and McGraw Hill Education, Maidenhead, pp. 25–41.

Lucas K., Lloyd B. (2005) *Health Promotion: Evidence and Experience*. Sage, London.

Marmot M., Wilkinson R. (eds) (2006) *Social Determinants of Health*, 2nd edn. Oxford University Press, Oxford.

Michie S., Rumsey N., Fussell A., Hardeman W., Johnston M., Newman S., Yardley L. (2007) *Improving Health: Changing Behaviour. NHS Health Trainer Handbook*. Department of Health, London, available at http://www.dh.gov.uk

National Institute for Health and Clinical Excellence (NICE) (2007) *Behaviour Change at Population, Community and Individual Levels*. NICE, London, available at http://www.nice. org.uk

Neighbourhood Renewal Unit (2003) *Updating the English Indices of Deprivation 2000 – Stage 2 'Blueprint' Consultation Report*. Office of the Deputy Prime Minister, London, available at http://www.neighbourhood.gov.uk

Neighbourhood Statistics (2008) available at http://neighbourhood.statistics.gov.uk/dissemina-tion/LeadPage.do?pageId=1001&tc=1205772919507&a=3&i=1001&m=0&s=1205772919 507&enc=1 (accessed 17 March 2008).

North F., Syme S., Feeney A., Shipley M., Marmot M. (1996) Psychosocial work environment and sickness absence among British civil servants: the Whitehall II study. *American Journal of Public Health* 86(3): 332–340.

Section 2

Nursing and Midwifery Council (NMC) (2007) Essential Skills Clusters (ESCs) for Pre-registration Nursing Programmes. NMC Circular 07 (2007) Annexe 2, available at http://www.ukcc.org.uk/aArticle.aspx?ArticleID=2914 (accessed 18 March 2008).

Nursing and Midwifery Council (NMC) (2008) *The Code: Standards of Conduct, Performance and Ethics for Nurses and Midwives.* Nursing and Midwifery Council, London.

Office for National Statistics (2008) *Super Output Areas,* available at http://www.ons.gov.uk/about-statistics/user-guidance/lm-guide/availability/sub-nat-lm/super-output-areas--soas-/index.html (accessed 22 November 2008).

Office of Public Sector Information (1998) *Public Interest Disclosure Act.* Available at http://www.opsi.gov.uk/acts/acts1998/ukpga_19980023_en_1#l1g1 (accessed 18 March 2008).

Olds D.L., Henderson C.R., Kitzman H.J., Eckenrode J.J., Cole R.E., Tatelbaum R.C. (1999) Pre natal and infancy visitation by nurses: recent findings. *The Future of Children* 9(1): 44–65.

Pearson P. (2003) Public health and health promotion. In: *Public Health in Policy and Practice: A Sourcebook for Health Visitors and Community Nurses* (ed. Cowley S.). Baillière Tindall, London, pp. 44–62.

Porter S. (1997) The patient and power: sociological perspectives on the consequences of holistic care. *Health and Social Care in the Community* 5(1): 17–20.

Rollnick S., Mason P., Butler C. (1999) *Health Behavior Change: A Guide For Practitioners.* Churchill Livingstone, London.

Ross C., Broh B. (2000) The roles of self esteem and the sense of personal control in the academic achievement process. *Sociology of Education* 73(4): 270–284.

Sandel M., Wright R. (2006) When home is where stress is: expanding the dimensions of housing that influence asthma morbidity. *Archives of Diseases in Childhood* 91: 924–948.

Shaw I. (2002) How lay are lay beliefs? *Health* 6(3): 287–299.

Skinner B.F. (1971) *Beyond Freedom and Dignity.* Penguin, Harmondsworth.

Wigley W. (2008) Quality and risk management: safeguarding children and vulnerable groups. In: *Public Health Skills, A Practical Guide for Nurses and Public Health Practitioners* (ed. Coles L., Porter L.). Blackwell, Oxford.

Wilkinson R.G. (2005) *The Impact of Inequality.* Routledge, London.

Wilkinson R.G., Kawachi I., Kennedy B.P. (1998) Mortality, the social environment, crime and violence. *Sociology of Health and Illness* 20(5): 578–597.

World Health Organisation (WHO) (1946) *WHO Constitution,* available at http://www.searo.who.int/LinkFiles/About_SEARO_const.pdf (accessed 15 March 2008).

Section 2

CHAPTER 9

Ethical and Legal Principles for Health Care

Stephen Richard Tee

Introduction

The purpose of this chapter is to help you appreciate and work within the ethical and legal frameworks that will impact on your practice as a nurse. Whilst not attempting to provide all the answers to every clinical situation, reading the chapter will help you navigate through ethical dilemmas, understand your legal obligations and support your professional development which in turn will assist your decision-making.

The specific learning outcomes addressed in this chapter, link with the Nursing and Midwifery Council's (NMC 2007) Essential Skills Clusters, and are identified below.

Learning outcomes

By the end of this chapter you will be able to do the following:

- Understand an ethical framework used to inform decision-making.
- Know and accept accountability and take appropriate responsibility.
- Work within legal frameworks for protecting self and others.
- Contribute to the planning of safe and effective care by appropriately recording and sharing information.

Nursing Ethics

Ethics involves consideration of the potential benefits and risks of taking decisions in practice. Nursing ethics reflects four broad areas of concern or what are known as ethical principles (McDonald 2001). First, respect for the person (*autonomy*), second, the obligation to maximise benefits (*beneficence*), third, to avoid harm and keep people safe (*non-maleficence*) and fourth, the responsibility to treat everyone equally and ensure that they are informed of their rights (*justice*).

The NMC's Code uses these principles to focus on the standards for conduct, performance and ethics (NMC 2008). The Code broadly adopts a *deontological perspective* which means it is based on the rights of the individual and the responsibilities or duties of the nurse. Deontology is sometimes known as 'duty'-based ethics and is discussed in more detail in Broad's (1930) book on ethical theory. The Code, summarised in Box 9.1, emphasises important values which are shared by all UK health care regulatory bodies.

Ethical Dilemmas

An ethical dilemma arises when there are clear ethical reasons both for and against taking a decision or a particular course of action (Pierce 1997). Nurses frequently encounter ethical dilemmas and so it is helpful to have strategies for managing such situations. Strategies should enable the nurse to recognise a dilemma, evaluate the options and take a decision. It is also important to reflect on or think about these decisions in order to further develop insight into the values which may have impacted on the decision the nurse has taken.

BOX 9.1

The Nursing and Midwifery Council (NMC 2008) *The Code: Standards of Conduct, Performance and Ethics for Nurses and Midwives*. Reproduced with the kind permission of the Nursing and Midwifery Council

The people in your care must be able to trust you with their health and well-being. To justify that trust, you must do the following:

- make the care of people your first concern, treating them as individuals and respecting their dignity;
- work with others to protect and promote the health and well-being of those in your care, their families and carers, and the wider community;
- provide a high standard of practice and care at all times; and
- be open and honest, act with integrity and uphold the reputation of your profession.

As a professional, you are personally accountable for actions and omissions in your practice and must always be able to justify your decisions.

You must always act lawfully, whether those laws relate to your professional practice or personal life.

Failure to comply with this Code may bring your fitness to practice into question and endanger your registration.

A helpful model, articulated by Erickson (1989), involves the nurse identifying four key aspects of any situation (ethical dilemma).

- Awareness of oneself
- Awareness of the situation
- Awareness of the professional perspective
- Awareness of the legislation.

If we break each of these aspects down further, *awareness of oneself* involves understanding one's own values. In other words, looking at sources of potential bias which may influence the decision you take. This can occur when your own values are in conflict with those of the patient. In ethical decision-making it is important to avoid letting one's own personal values from influencing decision-making, otherwise decisions taken may reflect the needs and priorities of the nurse rather than those of the patient.

Awareness of the situation involves such elements as knowledge of the clinical condition, social and legal status of the patient and the family circumstances. However, it also involves an appreciation of the spiritual and cultural values of the patient to ensure that the decisions taken are complementary rather than antagonistic to the patient's values and beliefs.

As previously discussed, *awareness of the professional perspective* is demonstrated in the NMC Code, which details the significant professional considerations and sets the parameters within which ethical professional practice can occur. In other words, many actions are prescribed by the Code such as the importance of cooperating with other members of the multidisciplinary team.

Finally the nurse cannot function safely and effectively without an *awareness of legislation*. Where a law forbids certain actions the situation is not an ethical dilemma, because the nurse may not have any other choice but to obey the law. These aspects are further developed through Activity 9.1.

Completing Activity 9.1 will have revealed the many dimensions to professional decision-making. To further explore these issues consideration will now be given to key professional and legal concepts which will have a direct impact on the professional behaviour of the practicing nurse.

Activity 9.1

Managing a dilemma

Think about a recent situation in practice where you felt there were good reasons both for and against a particular course of action. Then work through the following stages:

- What were your feelings about the situation?
- What were the clinical, social and family circumstances?
- Using the Code of Practice were there any specific professional considerations?
- Were there any specific legal considerations?
- What action was finally taken and do you think this was justified on all the grounds considered above?
- What would you do differently next time?

Accountability for Practice

Nursing is a complex human activity demanding the qualities of caring, sensitivity and self-awareness. Activity 9.1 illustrates how there are often many considerations when evaluating a course of action. As previously discussed, professional practice does not occur in a vacuum, but takes place within the context of legal and ethical obligations. Nurses are accountable for their practice and must be prepared to explain and justify their actions. Accountability in nursing remains an individual responsibility and so awareness of legal and professional regulation is an essential requirement for effective practice. It requires nurses to think carefully about the decisions they make and the actions they are going to take as a result of their decisions.

Governance – accountability within organisations

A broader but no less important dimension of accountability for the nurse to consider arises from the governance structures within the organisation in which the nurse works. Governance refers to the systems, controls and processes used in running the organisation. There are several forms of governance within the NHS which include Clinical Governance, Corporate Governance and Research Governance. However, more recently, the term Integrated Governance has emerged as the means by which these separate arrangements become streamlined, so that over time there can be greater integration between systems. It is increasingly important for NHS organisations to follow good business practices which ensure that they quickly introduce change where services need to be improved. Integrated Governance aims to achieve this through the following:

> Systems, processes and behaviours by which trusts lead, direct and control their functions in order to achieve organisational objectives, safety and quality of service and in which they relate to patients and carers, the wider community and partner organisations. (DH 2006a, p. 10)

It is therefore the means by which executives and non-executives ensure that the organisation is effective. The eight key elements of Integrated Governance are identified in Box 9.2.

Whilst all of these elements are important for organisational effectiveness, the most pertinent for the nurse, is number 5 which refers to Clinical Governance requirements. Clinical Governance is the system for improving standards of clinical practice. It was first defined in the 1998 consultation document, *A First Class Service: Quality in the New NHS* (DH 1998, p. 33), and by Scally and Donaldson (1998) as follows:

> A framework through which NHS organisations are accountable for continuously improving the quality of their services and safeguarding high standards of care by creating an environment in which excellence in clinical care will flourish.

Since 1998, the prominence of Clinical Governance has developed and remains central to modernised, patient-led health services and requires high levels of

---

BOX 9.2

Dimensions of Integrated Governance (from *Integrated Governance Handbook*, DH 2006a, p. 21) – The eight elements of Integrated Governance. Reproduced under the terms of the Click-Use Licence

1. Resources – be financially sustainable (probity, regularity, balance at year end), sufficient human resources, estate fit for purpose, appropriate information technology.
2. Efficiency and Economy, Effectiveness and Efficacy (4Es) – the organisation can be run effectively, efficiently, economically and challenged: why are we doing this activity, could someone else do it and do it better?
3. Compliance with authorisations – will be compliant at all times with its authorisation to operate (monitor, health & safety, drug and research management).
4. Compliance with Standards for Better Health and national targets – meet and exceed core standards and demonstrate progress with the developmental standards.
5. The duty of quality as reflected in Clinical Governance – continue to improve services for patients and be governed in accordance with current best practice.
6. The duty of partnership – cooperate with local health care economies.
7. The duty of patient and public involvement (Section 18 of the NHS Act) – have a growing and representative membership to which it is responsive and accountable, in particular, in the planning of services.
8. The ongoing development of the Board.

---

accountability for safe patient care. Whilst there have been different interpretations as to the meaning of Clinical Governance, for the nurse working in health care it is important to appreciate that it is not just a bureaucratic process but is fundamentally founded on concern for others (the ethical principle of deontology). The key components of Clinical Governance are identified in Box 9.3.

As we have seen, the NMC Professional Code and Clinical Governance arrangements within organisations make an important contribution to the context of modern nursing practice. Whilst there is clearly some overlap in their emphasis, in reality they take a different perspective on accountability for decisions taken. The NMC Code requires accountability to the professional body, whereas Clinical Governance demands accountability, through health organisations, to patients, the wider public, professional peers, colleagues and senior managers. In the event of a complaint about their behaviour, in areas such as the prevention of harm, the promotion of rights, maintenance of confidentiality or the production of health records, the nurse may be required to respond to two separate investigatory processes in explaining and justifying their actions.

For the nurse to be able to practice effectively within legal parameters and ensure that patients rights are protected, it is important to have a working knowledge of individual's rights both as a citizen and as a patient. The following sections explore each of these and also examine those aspects enshrined in law such as the *Human Rights Act* (Department of Constitutional Affairs 1998), *Data Protection Act* (1998) and the *Freedom of Information Act* (2000). It will also examine other 'rights' defined within policy initiatives including *The NHS Plan* (DH 2000) and codes of practice such as the *NHS Confidentiality Code of Practice* (DH 2003b) and *Standards on Records and Record Keeping* (NMC 2005).

BOX 9.3

Components of Clinical Governance (NHS Clinical Governance Support Team 2008, http://www.cgsupport.nhs.uk/About_CG/default.asp). Reproduced under the terms of the Click-Use Licence

- Patient, Public and Carer Involvement – Analysis of patient–professional involvement and interaction, and strategy, planning and delivery of care.
- Strategic Capacity and Capability – Planning, communication and governance arrangements and cultural behaviour aspects.
- Risk Management – Incident reporting, infection control, prevention and control of risk.
- Staff Management and Performance – Recruitment, workforce planning and appraisals.
- Education, Training and Continuous Professional Development – Professional re-validation, management development, confidentiality and data protection.
- Clinical Effectiveness – Clinical audit management, planning and monitoring, learning through research and audit.
- Information Management – Patient records and so on.
- Communication – Patient and public, external partners, internal, board and organisation-wide.
- Leadership – Throughout the organisation, including Board, Chair and non-executive directors, chief executive and executive directors, managers and clinicians.
- Team Working – Within the service, senior managers, clinical and multidisciplinary teams, and across organisations.

Activity 9.2

Promoting autonomy

Mary Ball is admitted to the assessment unit following referral by her GP. On admission Jenny, the nurse, introduces herself to Mary and takes her to a side room. Mary, who is feeling very anxious, is shown around the ward and asked to get into a hospital gown. Jenny then completes the admission notes and calls the doctor to complete the admissions process.

   Identify any actions the nurse could have taken in order to promote Mary's autonomy

Autonomy

Autonomy is an important concept in nursing, as it is about respect for another person's individuality and uniqueness. According to MacDonald (2002) autonomy has two elements to it, one reflecting the individual's capacity for taking their own decisions and another which demands that we do not interfere with the individual's control over their own lives. In other words we should, as nurses, wherever possible be actively seeking to create an environment where patients and clients can exercise autonomous decision-making. It is important to understand this principle otherwise our actions can inhibit a person's autonomy, see Activity 9.2.

It is clear from the scenario above that there are simple steps that a nurse can take to ensure Mary is fully informed and given as much control as possible over decisions. In such circumstances the nurse, whether he or she realises it or not, is in a very powerful position. Nurses have information about the environment and routines, they understand the technical jargon being spoken or which may be on display and, perhaps most importantly, they often have more knowledge of the person's condition, prognosis and treatment. In our efforts to promote autonomy it is easy to see how this power can be shared and used to empower Mary or can be withheld which will keep her in the dark and possibly increase her anxiety.

The culture of the ward environment is also important here as even when someone like Mary is capable of understanding the information, is fully informed, by Jenny, of the procedures and is not coerced by Jenny in any way, if the wider team is not committed to the promotion of independent decision-making then all Jenny's work will be quickly undone and Mary will start to feel disempowered. As MacDonald (2002) points out, the central issue is that those people using health and social care services have the ethical and legal right to have control over their own health care. We will now consider from where such 'rights' originate.

Human Rights Act 1998 (HRA98)

Whilst there are many pieces of legislation influencing almost all aspects of an individual's life, perhaps the most important of these is the *Human Rights Act* (1998) (HRA 1998a) which safeguards the rights of all UK citizens. The HRA98 came into full force in October 2000 and gives effect to the fundamental rights and freedoms contained within the European Convention on Human Rights.

The Department for Constitutional Affairs provides a clear outline of the HRA98 which, importantly for nurses, makes it unlawful for a public authority, like a government department, local authority or the police, to breach the Convention rights, unless an Act of Parliament meant it could not have acted differently. One example of this could be the use of mental health legislation to compulsorily admit someone to hospital in order to prevent harm to themselves or other people.

The 16 basic rights (listed in Box 9.4) are taken from the European Convention on Human Rights and set out important rights on issues of life and death as well as people's rights in everyday life.

What is the relevance of HRA98 to nursing?

It is not only important for the nurse to be aware of the convention on human rights but to also ensure that the convention guides actions and informs practice. The HRA98 states that all public authorities, including the National Health Service (NHS) and Local Authorities, should take account of people's rights when making decisions about the provision of services. The private and independent sector services are also covered by this provision where they are carrying out public functions.

As an employee of a public authority, nurses may have a direct influence over decisions taken in the name of the organisation. Nurses are often in the position of caring for people at vulnerable times in their lives. They may be participants in life and death decisions, have involvement with people's property and possessions, be exposed to different views and values to their own and be required to accommodate

---

BOX 9.4

A summary of the convention rights taken from *A Guide to the Human Rights Act* (1998) (HRA 1998b). For a more detailed explanation see http://www.dca.gov.uk/peoples-rights/human-rights/index.htm. Reproduced under the terms of the Click-Use Licence

RIGHT TO LIFE – The absolute right to have your life protected by law.

PROHIBITION OF TORTURE – The absolute right not to be tortured or subjected to treatment or punishment which is inhuman or degrading.

PROHIBITION OF SLAVERY AND FORCED LABOUR – The absolute right not to be treated as a slave or forced to perform certain kinds of labour.

RIGHT TO LIBERTY AND SECURITY – The right not to be deprived of your liberty – 'arrested or detained'– except in limited cases specified in the Article and where this is justified by a clear legal procedure.

RIGHT TO A FAIR TRIAL – The right to a fair and public hearing within a reasonable period of time.

NO PUNISHMENT WITHOUT LAW – The right not to be found guilty of an offence arising out of actions which at the time committed were not criminal.

RIGHT TO RESPECT FOR PRIVATE AND FAMILY LIFE – The right to respect for private and family life, home and correspondence.

FREEDOM OF THOUGHT, CONSCIENCE AND RELIGION – Freedom to hold a broad range of views, beliefs and thoughts, as well as religious faith.

FREEDOM OF EXPRESSION – The right to hold opinions and express views on alone or in a group.

FREEDOM OF ASSEMBLY AND ASSOCIATION – The right to assemble with other people in a peaceful way.

RIGHT TO MARRY – The right to marry and start a family. The national law will still govern how and at what age this can take place.

PROHIBITION OF DISCRIMINATION – The right not to be treated differently because of race, religion, sex, political views or any other status, unless this can be justified objectively.

PROTECTION OF PROPERTY – The right to the peaceful enjoyment of possessions.

RIGHT TO EDUCATION – The right not to be denied access to the educational system.

RIGHT TO FREE ELECTIONS – Elections for members of the legislative body (e.g. Parliament) must be free and fair and take place by secret ballot.

ABOLITION OF THE DEATH PENALTY – Protocol 13 replaced Protocol 6 and abolishes the death penalty in all circumstances.

---

difference in terms of faith, gender and race. There are many instances where the nurse could, through a thoughtless action or omission, inadvertently contravene the HRA98. Nurses must be vigilant in their practice to ensure that they, or the organisation for which they work, do not discriminate against individuals or act in ways which do not respect these fundamental human rights.

Patients' rights

In addition to the rights detailed in the HRA98, individuals also have rights as patients of the NHS in the United Kingdom. However, patient groups (Action Network 2007) have expressed concern that patients are not always fully informed of their rights. In America, the Government has gone a step further by introducing the *US Patients Bill of Rights* (President's Advisory Commission 1998) which clearly outlines a patient's rights and health organisation's obligations.

In the United Kingdom, to understand patient's rights it is important to understand the origins of the NHS. The NHS was established in 1948 with the three broad aims of meeting the needs of *everyone*, ensuring that services were free at the point of delivery and based on clinical need, rather than on the ability to pay (NHS Choices 2007). The individual rights of patients did not figure too highly in the way the NHS ran until the publication of the Patients Charter by John Major's Conservative Government in the 1990s. This was arguably the first real attempt to empower patients and inform them of what they should expect from the NHS. The Charter reflected the wider NHS policy drive of defining, in consumerist terms, the standards of public service to which patients were entitled.

Whilst at the time the Charter was seen as a positive development (Stocking 1991) the Charter had its critics with standards being seen as weak and unenforceable. With the arrival of the new Labour Government in 1997, the Patient's Charter was abolished as part of the introduction, in 2000, of the *NHS Plan*. The *NHS Plan* (DH 2000) was Labour's ten-year plan for the modernisation of the NHS and whilst not fundamentally changing individual rights it added some new principles which underpinned the provision of modernised services (see Box 9.5).

Once again there is a strong deontological theme running through these principles with an emphasis on the rights of users of services and the responsibilities of service organisations to provide some assurances of basic level of service provision. A further development has seen the introduction of the patient choice initiative which seeks to allow patients to choose where and when to have treatment from a list of hospitals and clinics. It includes local hospitals, NHS foundation trust hospitals and an increasing number of independent sector treatment centres contracted from the private sector to provide services to NHS patients.

The right to choose where and when to have treatment is an important transfer of power over the decision-making process which builds on existing rights. The issue of patient rights in the United Kingdom is controversial in that the rights

BOX 9.5

The NHS Plan core principles for a modernised NHS (DH 2000).
Reproduced under the terms of the Click-Use Licence

The NHS will do the following:

- Provide a universal service for all based on clinical need, not ability to pay.
- Provide a comprehensive range of services.
- Be based around the needs and preferences of individual patients, their families and their carers.
- Respond to the different needs of different populations.
- Work continuously to improve the quality of services and to minimise errors.
- Support and value its staff.
- Ensure that public funds for health care are devoted solely to NHS patients.
- Work with others to ensure a seamless service for patients.
- Help to keep people healthy and work to reduce health inequalities.
- Respect the confidentiality of individual patients and provide open access to information about services, treatment and performance.

Section 2

are somewhat limited. Whilst a full detailed description can be found on the *NHS Advice Guide* (Citizens Advice 2008) the following list (see Box 9.6) provides some examples of patients' rights. However, it also includes the limitations to these rights resulting in a reduced empowerment for the patient.

As can be seen it appears somewhat confusing for patients who are trying to determine their entitlements to the services of a GP. This can create considerable difficulties especially for the elderly and vulnerable. The same could also be said in the area of hospital treatment, as outlined in Box 9.7.

BOX 9.6

Patient's rights to NHS treatment from their general practitioner (GP) (adapted from *NHS Advice Guide*, Citizens Advice 2008). Reproduced from www.adviceguide.org.uk, with permission of Citizens Advice

- A UK citizen can choose his or her GP but the GP is not obliged to accept that person if there are reasonable grounds for not doing so. Their reasons must be supported in writing.
- Once registered the patient is entitled to treatment from a GP at the surgery where he or she is registered but the patient has no automatic right to see his or her own GP or to a home visit.
- Where a home visit is agreed it remains up to the GP to decide how urgently to visit. Patients can request a second opinion but the GP does not have to agree if the GP does not believe it unnecessary.
- Patients can however change their GP without having to provide justification and the local Primary Care Trust must provide details of how to go about this.
- A GP may be able to remove a patient from the patient register in some situations, for example, because the patient moves out of the practice area or is physically or verbally abusive to people at the practice.

BOX 9.7

Patient's 'rights' to NHS hospital care (adapted from *NHS Advice Guide*, Citizens Advice 2008). Reproduced from www.adviceguide.org.uk, with permission of Citizens Advice

- Where a patient attends an accident and emergency department he or she should be assessed immediately and should not have to wait for more than 4 hours between attending the A and E department and subsequent admission, treatment or discharge.
- Patients are entitled to urgent medical attention in an emergency but cannot receive routine NHS hospital treatment without being referred by a GP.
- Patients have the right to see a doctor competent to deal with their case but they have no right to see a particular consultant or doctor, although this can be requested.
- Where a patient is unable to receive the hospital treatment he or she needs immediately, they may have to go on a waiting list for which there are maximum waiting times. If necessary, treatment may be arranged in an alternative hospital to meet this guarantee.
- Patients should not be discharged from hospital until their care needs are assessed and arrangements made to ensure they receive necessary services when discharged.
- Patients unhappy with the arrangements for discharge may ask for a review of the decision.
- Where an operation is cancelled an alternative date within 28 days of the original date or sooner for life-threatening conditions should be offered.

Activity 9.3

Promoting patient's rights

You are a nurse working within a community setting with a new community of families who have recently arrived in the United Kingdom from Eastern Europe. What strategies should the nurse employ to ensure that these service users are aware of their rights and have access to the full range of NHS services?

Unfortunately many of these 'rights' are not enforceable by individuals. NHS organisations may suffer financial penalties if they do not meet some of these standards such as waiting times. Where there is evidence of negligence, individuals do have recourse to the law but in the case of these standards of service not being met it will be down to individuals to complain to the NHS organisation.

Whatever the status of these rights it is evident from the above that there is a significant role for the nurse in communicating to patients and raising awareness of these rights and others added in the future. Patients and the public have a right to detailed information on local health services, including the standards of quality and maximum waiting times, which can be obtained from many sources in the NHS. In addition, the Department of Health (DH 2003a) has produced a *Code of Practice* on openness in the NHS which states that patients should have access to available information about NHS services and policies, including information on standards under the *NHS Plan*. These issues are further explored through Activity 9.3.

Consent

It is essential for the practicing nurse to have a good understanding of the concept of informed consent and the information patients need to receive and understand in order to provide informed consent.

A helpful guide to consent is contained in the RCN (2005) publication, *Informed Consent in Health and Social Care Research: RCN Guidance for Nurses*. Whilst pertaining to research the guide illuminates the principles common to consent to care and treatment. A useful definition of informed consent is the following:

> an ongoing agreement by a person to receive treatment, undergo procedures or participate in research, after risks, benefits and alternatives have been adequately explained to them. (RCN 2005, p. 3)

All nurses must ensure that they obtain consent before providing treatment or care. However, consent can only be said to be *informed* when a patient fully understands the facts about the treatment or care he or she is about to receive. This means that the patients not only need to be in possession of relevant facts, at the time of consenting, but they also need the opportunity to process the information. As part of this process the nurse will need to use strategies to determine whether the patients are capable of understanding their treatment or whether their ability

---

BOX 9.8

Circumstances where patients may be examined or given treatment without consent (*NHS Advice Guide,* Citizens Advice 2008). Reproduced from www.adviceguide.org.uk, with permission of Citizens Advice

- Patients who have a notifiable disease
- Carriers of a notifiable disease
- Detained under mental health legislation
- Life is in danger and they are unconscious and cannot indicate their wishes
- A child who is a ward of court and the court decides that a specific treatment is in the child's interests
- A court or someone who has parental responsibility authorises treatment. However, a person whose treatment is authorised by a court must be given an opportunity to defend his or her case against treatment in court.

---

to process the information is limited by such problems as cognitive impairment or intoxication.

The concept of informed consent is a legal term and reflects the patient's right to receive information about his or her condition (RCN 2005). Achieving informed consent will ensure that patients are not deceived or coerced into accepting treatment or care. There are, however, situations where patients may be examined or given treatment without consent (see Box 9.8).

Obtaining consent requires the nurse to use clear and sensitive communication skills and whilst in many cases consent may be obtained orally it is considered good practice to ask the patient to sign a consent form. This would particularly apply to procedures or treatments which carry a high risk. Some instances of where signed consent would be appropriate are for general anaesthesia, surgery and certain forms of drug therapy.

Once consent has been obtained the nurse should clearly record in the patient's notes the process used for obtaining the oral or written consent. However, it is important to understand that a patient's signature may be invalidated if he or she was not fully informed of the nature of the treatment, the risks and potential consequences.

Continued consent

It is important for the nurse to not see consent as a one-off process. Informed consent should be an ongoing requirement to ensure patients continue to understand the care and treatment they are receiving and any changes to the information originally supplied. Consent for one aspect of care and treatment does not imply consent for a further procedure or form of treatment.

Implied consent

The concept of implied consent is by its very nature controversial. In fact, Aveyard (2002) suggests that nurses should be wary of relying on implied consent due to the difficulty of distinguishing between consent and compliance. There are many examples of where a nurse might assume implied consent by the patient's actions but the component of information-giving remains a crucial element within the process of obtaining implied consent. Otherwise, as Aveyard (2002) points out, nurses are at risk of providing treatment and care without the patient's consent.

Children

There are special considerations for children around the issue of consent. In the case of young people aged 16 or over, but under 18, they can give independent consent to their own treatment and it is not necessary to obtain the consent of a parent or guardian. However, if the young person is considered incapable of giving his or her own consent, perhaps because he or she has a severe disability, the parent's or guardian's consent must be obtained. The capability issue is an important consideration but, unfortunately, there is no single general test of capacity. The judgement of capability is made by the health professional and is decided on the merits of each case.

When a child under the age of 16 is considered incapable of understanding the treatment then parental consent or a court order is required, except in an emergency. In the event of refusal, treatment can still be administrated with a parent or guardian's consent or by a court order.

The Right to Die

The law relating to an individual's right to die is rather unclear. On the one hand, patients have the right to discontinue their treatment knowing that such an act may cause them to die. On the other, it remains illegal for a health professional to induce or hasten death either through omission or commission of treatment. Patients are encouraged to complete a legally binding advance directive, also known as a living will, which indicates a patient's wishes in the event they become too ill to give consent to medical treatment (Citizens Advice 2008).

Confidentiality

As well as being the expectation already outlined in NMC's Code (NMC 2008) the Department of Health (DH 2003a) has published the *NHS Confidentiality Code of Practice* (DH 2003b) which is a guide for anyone working in an NHS organisation. It focuses on the issue of confidentiality and consent to use patient health records.

It outlines the duty of confidence which it suggests is

> when one person discloses information to another in circumstances where it is reasonable to expect that the information will be held in confidence. (DH 2003a, p. 7)

The guide details a helpful model of practice (see Figure 9.1) detailing the components of a confidential service. The four key requirements are the following:

- Protect – clinicians must protect patient information
- Inform – service users must be made aware of how their information will be used

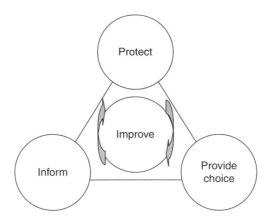

Figure 9.1   The confidentiality model (DH 2003a). Reproduced under the terms of the Click-Use Licence.

- Provide choice – the requirements to facilitate decision-making about whether confidential information can be disclosed or used in particular ways
- Improve – a continuous process of exploring better ways to protect, inform and provide choice.

The nurse's legal and professional obligations around the protection of confidential information are rather complex. Patients also have the right to confidentiality under the *Data Protection Act* 1998, the *Human Rights Act* 1998 and the common law duty of confidence. The legislation concerning health records will now be considered.

Health Records

To maintain the quality of care it is clearly essential to keep written health records which detail the care and treatment provided and future plans. Health providers have a duty to ensure these records are full and accurate, are secure and confidential and are written in an accessible format. It is considered good practice for nurses and other health professionals to agree what they are going to record about the patient, to provide copies of letters and, if asked, share what they have written.

In nursing, effective record keeping is a vital aspect of practice and one which, according to the NMC (2005), helps to support high standards of clinical care, maintain continuity of care, promote communication, ensure accuracy and detect changes in the patient's condition. In 2005, the NMC produced a revised version of their *Guidelines for Records and Record Keeping* (NMC 2005), which clearly details the expectations of the content and style of good record keeping (see Box 9.9).

> **BOX 9.9**
>
> **Summary advice on record keeping (NMC July 2007 advice@nmc-uk.org.). Reproduced with the kind permission of the Nursing and Midwifery Council**
>
> - Record keeping is an integral part of nursing, midwifery and specialist community public health nursing practice.
> - Good record keeping is a mark of a skilled and safe practitioner.
> - Records should not include abbreviations, jargon, meaningless phrases, irrelevant speculation, offensive or subjective statements.
> - Records should be recorded using terms that the patient or client can easily understand.
> - Auditing records can identify areas for staff training and development.
> - Registrants must ensure that any entry made in a record is easily identified.
> - Patients and clients have the right of access to records held about them.
> - Each practitioner's contribution to records should be seen as of equal importance.
> - Registrants have a duty to protect the confidentiality of the patient and client record.
> - The principles of confidentiality apply equally to computer and manually held records.
> - Local research ethics committee should approve the use of records in research.
> - Registrants must use their professional judgement to decide what is relevant and what should be recorded.
> - Records should be factual, consistent and accurate, written in a way that the meaning is clear.
> - Records should be recorded clearly and in such a manner that the text cannot be erased or deleted without a record of change.
> - Registrants need to assume that entries made in a patient or client record will at some point be scrutinised.
> - Good record keeping helps to protect the welfare of patients and clients.

Sharing information

Everyone has the right to request information held by public sector organisations under the *Freedom of Information Act* (FOI) 2000, which came into force in January 2005. Patients have the right to see most health records held about them, subject to certain safeguards. They are also entitled to be informed of how information about them will be used and how they can arrange to see their records. Patients can ask for copies of all records about themselves although they may have to pay a fee.

The FOI gives individuals the right to ask any public body for all information they have on any subject they choose and normally the organisation must provide the information within a month. This means that patients can request all personal information held about them. The FOI applies to all 'public authorities' including heath trusts, hospitals and doctors' surgeries. There are no restrictions on age or nationality as to who can request the information (although personal information will be handled under the *Data Protection Act* instead of the *Freedom of Information Act* – see below). Consequently, the FOI places an obligation on public authorities to manage their information in accordance with a publication scheme which describes the 'classes' or 'kinds' of information held.

> **BOX 9.10**
>
> **The Data Protection Principles (adapted from http://www.direct.gov.uk/en/ RightsAndResponsibilities/DG_10028507). Reproduced under the terms of the Click-Use Licence**
>
> The Data Protection Principles require personal information to be the following:
>
> - fairly and lawfully processed;
> - processed for limited purposes;
> - adequate, relevant and not excessive;
> - accurate;
> - not kept longer than necessary;
> - processed in accordance with your rights;
> - kept secure;
> - not transferred abroad without adequate protection.

Data Protection

The *Data Protection Act* (1998) establishes rules which prohibit the misuse of personal information by any organisation, known as 'data controllers', in the United Kingdom. The eight rules are known as the Data Protection Principles (see Box 9.10) and provide protection of sensitive personal data such as ethnicity, religious belief, trade union membership and sexual life.

The NHS Care Record guarantee

This guarantee for NHS Care Records in the United Kingdom (NHS 2005) provides a commitment that records will only be used in ways which respect patient's rights and promote their health and well-being. The guarantee aims to ensure that people who care for patients only use records to provide the basis for health care decisions, allow partnership in care decisions, ensure safety and effectiveness of care and enable effective inter-professional collaboration. It also guarantees that others in the NHS may only use records to check the quality of care through clinical audit, protect the health of the general public, keep track of spending, manage the health service, help investigate concerns or complaints, teach health care workers and help with research.

Protecting patient-identifiable information

To protect patient information the NHS and Social Services are required to appoint senior staff to the role of Caldicott Guardian (DH 2006b). Caldicott Guardians are senior staff, in NHS and Social Service organisations, appointed to protect patient information and were established in response to the 1997 report of the Review of Patient-Identifiable Information, chaired by Dame Fiona Caldicott. The review resulted in a number of recommendations aimed at

> regulating the use and transfer of patient-identifiable information between NHS organisations in England and to non-NHS bodies. (DH 2006b, p. 1)

The Caldicott Committee's remit included

> all patient-identifiable information passing between organisations for purposes other than direct care, medical research, or where there was a statutory requirement for information. The aim was to ensure that patient-identifiable information was shared only for justified purposes and that only the minimum necessary information was shared in each case. (DH 2006b, p. 1)

Caldicott Guardians are appointed by the Chief Executives of the NHS and Social Service organisations and a national register is maintained, on which there are approximately 750 registered Caldicott Guardians, working within the NHS, Social Care and other health-related organisations. A manual for Caldicott Guardians (DH 2006b) which explains their role and function can be found on the Department of Health website. In essence they are the 'Guardian' of person-based clinical information and overseer of the arrangements for the use and sharing of clinical information and must ensure systems and processes adhere to the following principles:

Principle 1 – Justify the purpose(s) for using confidential information
Principle 2 – Only use it when absolutely necessary
Principle 3 – Use the minimum that is required
Principle 4 – Access should be on a strict need-to-know basis
Principle 5 – Everyone must understand his or her responsibilities
Principle 6 – Understand and comply with the law.

The Caldicott Guardian is therefore a useful resource for the nurse in the event of having a query as to whether they can safely share information with others outside of their organisation (Activity 9.4).

Activity 9.4

Sharing information

An informal patient, Julia, who is being cared for on a mental health unit asks the nurse if she can read her medical and nursing notes. How should the nurse respond to Julia's request and what actions should the nurse take in order to meet Julia's needs for information?

Conclusion

As we have seen many of the codes and principles explored in this chapter adopt a common *deontological perspective*, emphasising both the rights of the individual, receiving health care, and the responsibilities or duties of professionals involved in delivering treatment and care. The dynamic context of practice arising from technological advances, policy initiatives and legislative developments, both within the United Kingdom and Europe, mean that new rights and responsibilities emerge with alarming frequency.

Section 2

This chapter has explored *current* legal and ethical frameworks which influence contemporary nursing practice but it remains incumbent on all registered nurses to maintain their knowledge of changes in this important area of practice, in order to protect the rights of patients in their care. It would therefore seem essential to develop lifelong learning strategies, such as attending mandatory training, accessing professional journals and visiting key websites (such as those listed in the reference list), so that practice reflects modern ethical frameworks and operates within the parameters of the law.

References

Action Network (2007) Available at http://www.bbc.co.uk/dna/actionnetwork/C2108

Aveyard H. (2002) Implied consent prior to nursing care procedures. *Journal of Advanced Nursing* 39(2): 201–207.

Broad C.D. (1930) *Five Types of Ethical Theory*. Harcourt Brace, New York.

Citizens Advice (2008) *NHS Advice Guide*. Available at http://www.adviceguide.org.uk/index/family_parent/health/nhs_patients_rights.htm

Data Protection Act (1998) Available at http://www.uk-legislation.hmso.gov.uk/acts/acts1998/ukpga_19980029_en_1

Department of Constitutional Affairs (1998) *A Guide to the Human Rights Act*. HMSO, London.

Department of Health (DH) (1998) *A First Class Service: Quality in the New NHS*. HMSO, London.

Department of Health (DH) (2000) *The NHS Plan: A Plan for Investment, a Plan for Reform*. The Stationery Office, London.

Department of Health (DH) (2003a) *Code of Practice on Openness in the NHS*. HMSO, London.

Department of Health (DH) (2003b) *NHS Confidentiality Code of Practice*. HMSO, London.

Department of Health (DH) (2006a) *Integrated Governance Handbook*. NHS, Department of Health, London.

Department of Health (DH) (2006b) *The Caldicott Guardian Manual*. Available at http://www.connectingforhealth.nhs.uk/systemsandservices/infogov/caldicott/caldresources/guidance/caldicott_2006.pdf

Erickson J. (1989) Steps to ethical reasoning. *The Canadian Nurse* August 23–24: 23–24.

Freedom of Information Act (2000) HMSO, London.

Human Rights Act (1998a) HMSO, London.

Human Rights Act (1998b) *A Guide to the Human Rights Act* (1998). Available at http://www.dca.gov.uk/peoples-rights/human-rights/index.htm

MacDonald C. (2002) Nurse autonomy as relational. *Nursing Ethics* 9(2): 194–201.

McDonald M. (2001) *A Framework for Ethical Decision-Making: Version 6.0 Ethics Shareware*. Available at http://www.ethics.ubc.ca/mcdonald/decisions.html

NHS Choices (2007) Available at http://www.nhs.uk/aboutnhs/HowtheNHSworks/Pages/about-thenhs.aspx

NHS Clinical Governance Support Team (2008) Available at http://www.cgsupport.nhs.uk

NHS: The Care Record Guarantee (2005) Available at http://www.connectingforhealth.nhs.uk/nigb/crsguarantee

Nursing and Midwifery Council (NMC) (2005) *Standards on Records and Record Keeping.* NMC, London.

Nursing and Midwifery Council (NMC) (2007) *Essential Skills Clusters.* NMC Circular 07(2007) Annexe 2, NMC, London.

Nursing and Midwifery Council (NMC) (2008) *The Code: Standards of Conduct, Performance and Ethics for Nurses and Midwives.* Nursing and Midwifery Council, London.

Pierce P. (1997) What is an ethical decision? *Critical Care Nursing Clinic of North America* 9(1): 1–11.

President's Advisory Commission (1998) The President's Advisory Commission on Consumer Protection and Quality in the Health Care Industry. *Quality First: Better Health Care for All Americans.* US *Patients Bill of Rights.* Final Report to the President of the United States. Washington, DC. Available at http://www.hcqualitycommission.gov/final/append_a.html

Royal College of Nursing (RCN) (2005) Informed consent in health and social care research. *RCN Guidance for Nurses.* Available at http://www.rcn.org.uk/__data/assets/pdf_file/0010/78607/002267.pdf

Scally G., Donaldson L.J. (1998) Clinical governance and the drive for quality improvement in the new NHS in England. *British Medical Journal* 317: 61–65.

Stocking B. (1991) Patients charter – new rights issue. *British Medical Journal* 303: 1148–1149.

Section 2

Section 3

Infection Prevention and Control

Chapter 10 Precepts of Infection Prevention and Control
Joan Cochrane

CHAPTER 10

Precepts of Infection Prevention and Control

Joan Cochrane

In the face of intense and immediate crisis, when an outbreak of plague implanted fear of imminent death in an entire community, ordinary routines and customary restraint broke down. Rituals arose to discharge anxiety and local panic often provoked bizarre behaviour. The first effort at ritualizing responses to the plague took extreme and ugly forms.

(*Plagues and Peoples*, McNeill 1976, p. 133)

Introduction

Infection control is the responsibility of *everyone* who works within health care systems (Department of Health (DH) 2006a). In this chapter the theories that underpin high-quality infection control practice will be explored. The intention is to enable you to understand the theoretical components and how to adopt these into your everyday practice. It is anticipated that your current thinking about infection control will be challenged and in doing so, you will have a more informed perspective on this speciality.

The specific learning outcomes addressed in this chapter link with the Nursing and Midwifery Council's (NMC 2007) Essential Skills Clusters, and are identified below.

Learning outcomes

By the end of this chapter you will be able to do the following:

- Identify the need for risk assessment to prevent and control infections.
- Have an understanding of the standard principles for infection prevention and control practice.
- Develop knowledge into reducing infection risks when handling clinical waste, sharps, linen and body fluid spillages.

- Develop awareness of the need to maintain professional standards by promptly complying with the national and local policies and procedures to prevent and control spread of infection.
- Understand the principles of asepsis when undertaking clinical interventions.
- Develop an awareness of health promotion strategies that impact on the need to ensure public and patient safeguards against infection.

Modern Infection Control

The reality of the real world is that we are human beings and as such we are capable of infecting one another, sometimes unintentionally (Holland 2007). Infections do not recognise the social, political or organisational boundaries that society constructs, and in the healthy individual we have physiological mechanisms that enable us to fight infection. Within modern health care environments, infection control is the responsibility of all health care workers (HCWs) (Pratt *et al.* 2007). Remember that you have chosen this profession and you should endeavour to practice in a safe and competent manner (Healey & Spencer 2008).

In clinical practice we have everyday clinical decisions and moral and ethical deliberations to consider, as we strive to provide our patients with an environment that is microbiologically safe (Cochrane 2000). If our behaviours and clinical practices are of a low standard, then morally and ethically we are not fulfilling the NMC's Code (NMC 2008) or minimising harm to the patients. Disciplinary action may result from our lack of competence or negligence in our maintenance of infection control principles for clinical practice (DH 2006a).

The political, public and media attention focused upon infection control practice and the complexity of modern health care requires a need to be explicit in our attempts to assure everyone that we are safe, effective and competent practitioners in preventing and controlling the transmission of infection.

You can only be a safe practitioner if you are not only equipped with essential clinical skills, but also have an understanding of, and apply everyday, the theoretical knowledge that underpins those skills (Horton & Parker 2002).

Beginning the Journey

It is impossible to equip you, in one chapter, with all the theoretical knowledge needed around infection control practice; an overview of current evidence and standards for best practice is provided, to guide you in the acquisition of the requisite fundamental clinical skills. In tandem with your clinical placements, further academic and professional reading and course work, it is anticipated that your practice will be more informed, enabling you to adopt an inquisitive approach to care interventions. Similarly in a previous chapter, health promotion is addressed. You should reflect upon this now in order to determine those *health promotion strategies* you should employ when implementing infection control practices into your day-to-day activities. It may be helpful to read Chapter 8 – Promoting Health and Well-being – particularly the sections on Promoting Health and Well-being and Nursing and Health Behaviour Change Framework.

Activity 10.1

It is essential to have an understanding of microorganisms and their classification. Before reading any further answer the following questions:

- Are all microorganisms infectious?
- Identify the beneficial microorganisms and why they are of benefit to the human body?

Consider some of the microorganisms that you have encountered in providing patient care.

- What implications do these have for practice?
- How do microorganisms enter the body?
- How do the body defences resist or fight infection?
- Can you identify the clinical signs of infection?
- What is the chain of *infection?*
- How can the links in the chain be broken?

To help you begin the journey, this chapter is divided into the following themes:

- Identifying risks for infection
- Standard principles for infection control
- Standard isolation precautions
- Application of asepsis into clinical practice
- Managing waste, linen and spillages of blood or body fluids.
- Infection control and health promotion.

Before reading any further you should now undertake Activity 10.1.

Identifying Risks for Infection

The definition of risk is 'the possibility of suffering harm or loss; danger; the chances that a hazard will give rise to harm' (Thistlethwaite & Tie 2007). In examining health promotion theories Rogers (1985) is often cited, as he developed the Protection Motivation Theory (PMT). Infection control practice has a protection component within its framework. Rogers's work demonstrates how we can acquire transferable knowledge across the spectrum of health care when undertaking health promotion activity. After all you can only safeguard against risks if you know what those risks are.

Rogers's work suggested that health risk messages discussed the following:

- the probability that a threat would occur;
- the magnitude of anxiousness if a threat occurred; and
- the effectiveness of the recommended response to avert the threat.

Infection prevention and control embraces these three messages, in that we know that there are microorganisms that can cause infection, we need to protect staff, patients and visitors if an infection occurs and seek to employ mechanisms to control the spread of an infection.

Section 3

Microorganisms are invisible to the naked eye, and have the potential to cause harm in a susceptible human (Keyworth 2000, p. 19). In order for an infection to occur Orme *et al.* (2003) state that the following must exist:

- a *host* (a human who has been exposed to the harmful agent and who is *susceptible* to developing the infection)
- the *pathogen* (this may be bacteria, viruses or other infectious agents including chemicals)
- the *environment*, that is the pathway or vehicle for the infectious agent to cause harm.

Who is at risk?

The fact that a patient is receiving health care interventions, no matter how minor, can mean that they are *susceptible* to an infection, by virtue of them having an illness or disease. This in itself can lower patient immunity to disease or infection. A comprehensive, patient-associated risk assessment can be found in Horton and Parker (2002). See Activity 10.8 if you would like to explore this further.

The *age* of the patient is important as infection risks increase in the very young and the older person. In infants the immune system's mechanisms are not fully developed and in the older person the immune system's efficacy has begun to decline.

Patient well-being (both physiological and psychological), particularly if the patient's nutritional status is poor, as this can affect the body's ability to fight infection.

Underlying disease – patients may have a pre-existing condition, for example chronic pulmonary disease, neoplasm, diabetes or another infection and this can increase the risk of infection as the immune system may have been depressed.

Clinical interventions – patients have invasive medical devices and surgical procedures and any range of pharmacological interventions. All of these procedures can again increase the patient's susceptibility to infection.

Managing risk

Risk assessment for infection should be included in patient assessment and decisions in treatment and care of patients. Identified risks from an infection control perspective must be *documented* in the patient records. Staff can also be at risk of infection or transference of pathogens if they do not comply with good infection control practices.

Infection control has national standards for good practice (Pratt *et al.* 2007). While these standards are research/evidenced based, a lot of principles applied in infection control are also based on empirical knowledge (experience and observation) (Ayliffe *et al.* 2000). The combination of this researched-evidence and empirical knowledge, applied into day-to-day clinical practice, seeks to prevent the chances of an infection being transmitted from a *source* (e.g. person, contaminated equipment and so on).

All NHS hospitals, many Primary Care Trusts (PCTs) and increasingly other health care providers, have a dedicated *infection control team*. They will have the *expertise*

Activity 10.2

In your clinical environment identify who the members of the infection control team are and how to contact them?

---

and *specialist knowledge* to guide practice in the event of an infectious agent or infection being identified within the health care environment (Activity 10.2).

Patients and their visitors should also be made aware of any infection risks associated with their health care. This will enable them to make *informed choices* and to also comply with staff recommendations and adopt precautions that may safeguard themselves, staff and significant others. This education can be time-consuming, and may require a *collaborative* approach from not only immediately located staff, but also input from the infection control *specialist practitioners*.

All NHS organisations are required to have *infection control policies* and protocols that are supported by contemporary evidence. You must acquaint yourself with their location, and endeavour to read them.

Standard Principles for Infection Control Practice

In 2007, the updated 'epic' *guidelines* for preventing health care associated infections (HCAI) were published (Pratt *et al*. 2007). These National Guidelines provide updated recommendations for practice that reflects new evidence that has emerged since the original guidelines were published (Pratt *et al*. 2001). For *community practitioners*, the 'epic' team also produced complementary guidelines, pertinent to community and primary care practice (National Institute for Clinical Excellence (NICE) 2003). Systematic review of the best available evidence is included within both these guidelines, and it is this evidence that underpins a high standard of practice. You may hear practitioners refer to these guidelines as 'Universal Precautions'; this is the old terminology. Universal Precautions were rebranded as Standard Precautions for Infection control, in 1998, by the Centre for Disease Control (CDC) in Atlanta. This was due to combining the elements of universal precautions with body substance isolation precautions to have a more comprehensive and robust set of standardised guidelines for practice.

In England, the 'epic' guidelines must be adopted by all HCWs when providing care for all patients. The guidelines themselves do not address *specialist requirements* for some areas of practice, for example perioperative environment or occasions where outbreaks of infection occur, but they do include four distinct areas for best practice:

- Hospital environmental hygiene
- Hand hygiene
- Personal protective equipment
- The safe use and disposal of sharps.

These guidelines also provide guidance on *intravenous* and *urinary* catheter placement and management.

Hospital environmental hygiene

The world is full of *microorganisms* and the healthy individual usually lives in harmony with these. However, while many microorganisms do not cause a problem to humans, there are those that are pathogenic (i.e. cause disease). In recent years, associations have been made between HCAI and a poor level of hospital environmental hygiene (Dancer 1999; DH 2004, 2006b).

Pathogens responsible for HCAI have been widely found in hospital environments (Denton *et al.* 2004). These pathogens can be found on many surfaces and as these surfaces are touched by hands, these pathogens can be *transferred* to other surfaces or patients. It is essential that good hand hygiene practices are adopted by everyone in a health care environment (this should also include patients and their visitors).

Exogenous transmission of infection occurs when pathogens come into direct or non-direct contact with the patient (*cross-infection*). An example of direct contact would be where a patient is provided with a commode that has not been decontaminated following previous use. Similarly, indirect contact could occur if hands are not decontaminated prior to patient contact or a clinical activity.

Hospital environments must be visibly clean, be free from dust and dirt and be acceptable to patients, staff and visitors (Pratt *et al.* 2007). Environmental hygiene is not just about household cleaning and decontamination of equipment, within that environment, but also encompasses housekeeping, linen management, food and kitchen hygiene, safe collection of clinical and general waste and its subsequent disposal.

Hand hygiene

Maintaining good hand hygiene standards involves not only the techniques of decontamination, but also the need to critically examine the thinking involved in undertaking this activity (see Activity 10.3). An important guiding principle is that of providing safe, clean care to our patients (DH 2006b).

Hand decontamination is a low-tech clinical intervention that can prevent transmission of infection (DH 2006b). Surely in today's health care provision it is more economically beneficial to adopt a low-tech activity? Any non-compliance with this basic activity results in a breach in our 'Duty of Care' (NMC 2008). This in turn could result in the expensive, high-tech patient care procedures/interventions necessary to control and manage infection (Cochrane 2003).

Unclean hands have been shown to be a significant vehicle for the transmission of microorganisms and can contribute to outbreaks of infection in health care environments (Pratt *et al.* 2007). Decontaminating hands prior to a clinical intervention or activity can significantly reduce cross-infection (Pratt *et al.* 2007).

Activity 10.3

Consider yourself to be *the patient* – ask yourself 'where have that practitioner's hands been before they touched me?'

As a practitioner, what activities have you undertaken using your hands in the last hour? How often did you wash those hands?

Section 3

Decontamination of hands is a process for physically removing, destroying or reducing the number of transient and resident microorganisms on the skin surfaces of the hands (Ayliffe *et al.* 2000). Hands should be decontaminated between patients and between different care activities (Pratt *et al.* 2007).

National and international guidance on hand decontamination is based on research into the use of soap and water, alcohol-based products and antiseptic hand washing agents (Pratt *et al.* 2001). The choice of hand decontamination agent should be based upon an assessment of the activity. No artificial nails, nail polish, stoned rings or wrist watches should be worn and cuts and abrasions must be covered prior to decontaminating hands (Pratt *et al.* 2007). Organisational policies on dress code and hand hygiene will reflect this (Activity 10.4).

The technique of hand washing to render hands socially clean is demonstrated in Figure 10.1 (Ayliffe *et al.* 2000). This technique applies to the use of soap and

---

Activity 10.4

With the help of your mentor, access and read your organisation's dress code and hand hygiene guidelines.

The following technique is recommended and need only take 20 seconds.

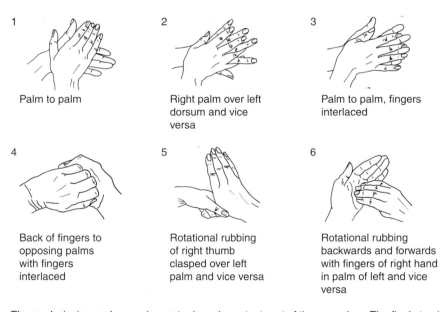

1 — Palm to palm

2 — Right palm over left dorsum and vice versa

3 — Palm to palm, fingers interlaced

4 — Back of fingers to opposing palms with fingers interlaced

5 — Rotational rubbing of right thumb clasped over left palm and vice versa

6 — Rotational rubbing backwards and forwards with fingers of right hand in palm of left and vice versa

Thorough rinsing under running water is an important part of the procedure. The final step is to dry the hands thoroughly using a paper towel for each hand – this not only prevents soreness, but also further reduces the number of transient bacteria that may still be present after hand washing.

Figure 10.1   Hand washing technique. Reproduced from Ayliffe G.A.J., Fraise A.P., Geddes A.M., Mitchell K. (eds) (2000) *Control of Hospital Infection: A Practical Handbook*, Copyright 2000 by permission of Edward Arnold (Publishers) Ltd.

water and also for alcohol-based agents. All surfaces of the hands must be covered. When using soap and water the actual physical activity of rubbing skin surfaces together and drying with paper towels reduces transient and resident bacterial counts. Similarly, when using an alcohol-based product, while this too reduces bacterial counts, the product must be allowed to dry (Pratt *et al.* 2007).

Remember that alcohol-based products should only be used *on* physically clean hands and these products are *not* sporicidal, therefore they will be ineffective against spore-forming organisms, for example *Clostridium difficile*. Current guidelines recommend washing hands with soap and water after repeated use of alcohol products (Pratt *et al.* 2007).

Personal protective equipment

Wearing uniforms or protective personal clothing is affected by current legislation (*Health and Safety at Work Act* 1974; National Health Service Executive (NHSE) 1995; Health and Safety Commission 2002; DH 2006a). Using protective equipment (PPE) will also reduce the risk of acquiring contamination from potentially infectious body fluids, and transmitting microorganisms via hands or clothing.

Throughout your clinical placements you will encounter many clinical practitioners and professionals allied to medicine (PAMs), in many health care environments, who do not wear uniform. Regardless of whether a uniform is worn or not, guidance and policies exist regarding the purchase of suitable attire, the laundry requirements of clothing and uniforms and a dress code policy (DH 2007; Pratt *et al.* 2007). In these instances, PPE is essential to protect the patient, the HCW and the environment from the possible carriage of pathogens on clothing.

As a student nurse, you will be issued with several pieces of uniform. Just as you considered in the previous section, where your hands had been prior to patient contact, also consider where your uniform has been. Wherever possible, do not wear uniform outside of hospitals or health care facilities, although we appreciate this is not always possible on community placements. Many organisations do not provide uniform laundry facilities and in this instance you should adhere to the current guidelines on washing uniforms separate from other items of household laundry (DH 2007).

The decision to wear PPE must be made following an assessment of the risks associated with a specific patient care intervention or activity.

Disposable aprons are single-use items. They are water repellent and impervious to microorganisms. Disposable aprons should be worn for all direct care procedures with patients when there is a likelihood of contact with blood, secretions, excretions or body fluids (Pratt *et al.* 2007). Similarly, aprons should be worn when handling linen, used equipment or waste products (Wilson 2001). Aprons should only be used for one procedure or one episode of care (Pratt *et al.* 2007). Infection control teams will advise when *gowns* should be worn (Pratt *et al.* 2007).

The wearing of *gloves* is not an alternative to hand decontamination. *Prior* to and *following* glove use, hands must still be washed or an alcohol-based agent applied.

Gloves will offer protection to your hands from possible contamination. There is concern around some glove materials causing sensitivity and adverse reactions

(Pratt *et al.* 2007) However, as with other items of PPE, the wearing of gloves and selection of the appropriate glove material must be made following a risk assessment.

This assessment should include the following: should gloves actually be necessary if a no-touch aseptic technique can be applied? (CDC 2007); should the gloves be sterile or non-sterile? The risks associated with any possibility of contact with secretions, body fluids and so on, or contact with non-intact skin or mucous membranes during the activity (Pratt *et al.* 2007). When gloves are worn with other PPE, they should be put on last (CDC 2007).

Gloves should always be discarded after every intervention or activity to prevent transmission of any microorganisms that they have come into contact with (Horton & Parker 2002).

Facemasks and eye protection are not always necessary for most nursing interventions. However, when there is the likelihood of accidental splashes from blood, body fluids, secretions and excretions to the face they must be worn (Arrowsmith 2005, p. 81; Pratt *et al.* 2007).

Specialised masks will be used when providing care for patients with specific respiratory diseases, for example tuberculosis (TB), Severe Acute Respiratory Syndrome (SARS) and so on (Pratt *et al.* 2007). Using these types of facemasks protects against inhalation of minute airborne particles, and ordinary surgical masks will not afford much protection against these particles. Your infection control team will provide advice when providing care to patients with specific infection control requirements as this type of mask needs to be specially fitted (Pratt *et al.* 2007).

If face protection is not worn, you may be exposed to *conjunctival* or *mucosal splashes* from blood or body fluids. In the event of this occurring you must follow the current policy in your area. See Box 10.1 for an example.

The safe use and disposal of sharps

Sharps are items that can cut or puncture the skin, for example needles, lancets, intravenous cannulae, bone fragments and sharp instruments. It is imperative that sharps are handled and disposed of correctly in relation to not only preventing cross-infection (through sharps or needle-stick injury) but also in maintaining

---

BOX 10.1

Policy example for exposure to conjunctival or mucosal splashes

- *Rinse* the area immediately with copious amounts of running water.
- Follow the guidance in *local policy* for this type of injury.
- *Report* the injury to your manger.
- Complete incident/accident *documentation.*
- *Identify* the source patient if possible.
- *Report* to occupational health immediately (or accident and emergency department if it is outside normal working hours) where a risk assessment will be undertaken and advice around post-exposure prophylaxis may be required.
- *Follow up* – comply with medical advice.

a safe environment. It is the responsibility of the person using the sharp to ensure that it is disposed of correctly (Arrowsmith 2005).

Sharps containers are now colour-coded, and this is discussed in the subsection on Health care waste of this chapter..

Patients who have a blood-borne virus (hepatitis B, hepatitis C or Human Immunodeficiency Virus (HIV)) may be unaware that they carry a blood-borne disease.

Safe practice with sharps is standardised in national and international guidelines to avoid needle-stick injuries (Box 10.2).

Needle protection devices are increasingly being introduced into clinical practice. Using these devices will enable safer working practices and assist in avoiding needle-stick or sharps injury. In the event of a needle-stick injury occurring, you should take immediate remedial action and also consult your local policy. It is your responsibility in tandem with that of your manager to ensure that all procedures are carried out (Box 10.3).

BOX 10.2

Safe practice with sharps (Pratt *et al.* 2007)

- *Never* pass sharps directly from hand to hand.
- *Never* bend or break a needle prior to disposal.
- *Do not* disassemble needles and syringes by hand prior to disposal. Never resheath a needle.
- *Always* take a sharps container to the patient.
- *Never* put fingers into a sharps container.
- *Always* use a sharps container that conforms to UN 3291 and BS 7320 at the point of use.
- *Always* assemble a sharps container according to the manufacturer's instructions and *complete* the security and disposal label.
- *Do not* fill the sharps container above the full indicator line.
- *Always* locate sharps containers in a safe position.

BOX 10.3

Immediate remedial action following needle-stick injury

- *Bleed* the puncture site.
- *Wash* the injury with soap and water.
- *Cover* the wound with a waterproof dressing.
- *Report* the injury to your manger.
- Complete incident/accident *documentation*.
- *Identify* the source patient if possible.
- *Report* to occupational health immediately (or accident and emergency department if it is outside normal working hours) where a risk assessment will be undertaken and advice around post-exposure prophylaxis may be required.
- *Follow up* – if required attend any follow-up testing.
- Counselling may be required.
- *Comply* with any advice given.

Standard Isolation Precautions

Technological advances in clinical interventions and surgical techniques in today's health care environment provide patient populations who are often critically ill and therefore susceptible to infection. Similarly, increased travel opportunities and shorter journey times enable many infections and communicable diseases to become pandemic in a very short space of time for example Severe Acute Respiratory Syndrome (SARS).

Standard principles for infection control are required for all patients at all times (Pratt *et al.* 2007), but patients known to have an infection (source) or be highly susceptible to infection need to be isolated from other patients to prevent transmission of infection.

Prior to isolating a patient, a comprehensive assessment needs to be undertaken that should include the *microbiology* and *epidemiology* of the organism and its *mode of transmission*.

Isolation techniques can sometimes be complex dependent upon the infectious agent. The CDC in Atlanta (2007) recently published new comprehensive guidelines for isolation. See Activity 10.8 if you would like to explore the web link to this site.

Source isolation is defined as the measures taken to prevent the spread of an infectious agent from an infected patient.

Protective isolation is utilised to protect those patients who are highly susceptible to developing an infection due to their suppressed immune system (Arrowsmith 2005).

Isolation is used for those infective microorganisms that are airborne (e.g. pulmonary tuberculosis, measles, chickenpox) and involves physical separation from other patients (Ayliffe *et al.* 2000).

Infected patients are housed in a single room with the door closed. These rooms often have air extraction (*negative pressure*) maintaining a flow of air into the room thus preventing contaminants and pathogens from reaching the surrounding environment. Health care facilities often do not have a large number of single isolation rooms, and in the event of several patients being infected or colonised with the same microorganism, then they may be nursed together in the same area. This is referred to as *cohort isolation.*

Patients in *protective isolation* should be in a single room with the door closed. The room may have *positive pressure* ventilation where air flows *out* of the room thus protecting the patient from pathogens and contaminants that might otherwise enter. Technological advances in ventilation systems often find patients needing protective isolation being cared for in high efficiency particulate air (HEPA) filtration rooms. These rooms have numerous air changes every hour to again significantly reduce the number of potential pathogens in the room.

Whichever type of isolation is being used, staff and visitors should be made aware of special precautions being in place, usually being informed by a *notice* at room entrance, observe strict *hand decontamination* on entering and leaving the room, wear *protective clothing* and be *highly compliant* with the standard principles for infection control (Wilson 2001). All health care organisations should have an isolation policy and the infection control team will be the first

Section 3

point of contact for specialist advice on what exact measures need to be adopted for individual infections.

Application of Asepsis into Clinical Practice

Asepsis is a state of being free from microorganisms (Hart 2007). In other words when we use an aseptic technique we are preventing sepsis occurring.

It is a technique that involves using equipment and fluids that are sterile during many clinical procedures or when managing certain clinical conditions, for example surgical wounds, fresh skin breaks, immunocompromised patient care, urinary and venous catheters (including peripheral cannulae) and other invasive clinical procedures including vaginal delivery in midwifery practice. It is also used for wounds that are healing by 'primary intention' (i.e. before the skin surface has sealed completely) (Wilson 2001).

In some chronic wounds the term 'healing by secondary intention' may be applied. These wounds are usually ulcers or pressure sores of long standing, some burns and some surgical wounds. With these wounds a 'clean' technique may be appropriate. Wound management texts will provide you with more knowledge on the healing process of wounds.

Once again an *assessment* must be undertaken to determine if the dressing requires a 'clean' technique or an aseptic technique. An example given by Wilson (2001) is for the removal of sutures, where a clean technique may be all that is required. Again assessment for wound dressings and implementing clinical interventions with medical devices such as intravascular devices must be documented. This enables reflection on an incident if sepsis occurs when used in conjunction with a root cause analysis tool (National Patient Safety Agency (NPSA) 2006).

Your hands are not sterile, and you may see forceps being used (known as a *no-touch* technique). Good hand decontamination and gloving technique assist in preventing cross-contamination (Arrowsmith 2005). No-touch technique is used when you do not want your hands coming into contact with the patient or the sterile equipment for example during catheterisation (Arrowsmith 2005). However, forceps can be difficult to manipulate and washing hands and using sterile gloves often affords better dexterity than forceps (Wilson 2001).

Surgical wound dressings should not be disturbed for 48 hours following the surgical procedure. This prevents possible endogenous infection from the bacteria present on the surrounding skin (Ayliffe *et al.* 2000). Wound dressings should only be removed when there is a clinical indication to do so, for example excessive wound exudate (Activity 10.5).

Activity 10.5

During your programme of study, you should practice the skills of aseptic techniques within the skills laboratory. If you do this with a colleague you can critique each other's technique. This will afford you opportunities to become proficient in opening sterile packs without contaminating any of the equipment and also allow you to practice your hand decontamination and gloving techniques.

Managing Waste, Linen and Spillages of Blood or Body Fluids

Health care waste

With the global environmental impact of disposing of waste, not to mention the need to reduce costs, there is a lot of legislation with which generators of health care waste have to comply (DH 2006c). If you work in Scotland or other countries within the European community, different classifications or rules may apply when segregating and disposing of health care waste.

The DH (2006c) document is very comprehensive and includes not only waste generated by acute hospitals but also guidance for community practitioners. The guidance approaches waste management by beginning with the segregation of waste using a colour-coded scheme. It also provides definitions for health care waste, infectious waste, medicinal waste and offensive/hygiene waste (Royal College of Nursing (RCN) 2007).

Segregation of waste is important as different types of waste pose different hazards. Segregation is undertaken by the person generating the waste.

All health care waste, irrespective of where it is generated is assumed to be infectious waste until it is assessed by the health care practitioner. Failure to segregate health care waste means that the whole waste stream has to be classified as infectious waste, which results in specialist handling, removal and increased organisational costs (DH 2006c).

Clinical waste is divided into two categories: that which poses a *risk of infection* and *medicinal waste*.

Infectious waste is that which poses a known or potential infection risk. This includes minor infections. Infectious waste also includes implanted medical devices that have been in contact with body fluids.

Medicinal waste includes unused and expired pharmaceutical products, drugs, vaccines, connecting tubing, bottles or boxes contaminated with pharmaceutical products, syringe bodies and drug vials. Controlled drugs are classified as non-cyto medicines and there are authorised personnel to whom their destruction or disposal should be referred (RCN 2007).

Hazardous waste is the classification applied to cytotoxic and cytostatic medicines.

Offensive/hygiene waste is classified as being non-clinical waste, that which is non-hazardous and non-infectious. This waste however could be offensive to those who come into contact with it. This type of waste includes incontinence and other waste produced from personal human hygiene, sanitary waste and nappies.

Colour coding facilitates the segregation of waste into different streams and ensures that each colour stream will be linked to the appropriate disposal path for that stream. Colour coding is outlined in a detailed chart within the DH (2006b) document.

Activity 10.6

With the help of your mentor make sure you are totally familiar with the colour-code system in your area of practice.

Colour-coded sharps containers facilitate the segregation of sharps ready for disposal as follows:

- *Yellow/orange lid* – for sharps *not* contaminated with medicinal products *or* fully empty sharps contaminated with medicinal products other than cyto-medicines. This waste is treated to render it safe prior to disposal.
- *Yellow/yellow lid* – for sharps which include sharps containing residual medicines or partially containing residual medicines. These containers require disposal by incineration.
- *Yellow/purple lid* – for waste that is contaminated with cytotoxic and cytostatic medicinal products. This waste is incinerated.

All clinical waste *should be labelled* with the point of origin. This enables traceability should problems arise during disposal (Wilson 2001; DH 2006c) (Activity 10.6)

Linen

Linen is not classified as clinical waste, but it still requires diligence with handling, segregation and disposal. Used linen can become contaminated from patients with microorganisms and body fluids. *Protective clothing* should be worn when handling linen (Pratt *et al.* 2007). Different types and colour coding of linen bags is used for linen segregation and this assists in determining the laundry process (i.e. the water temperature) required for the linen contained within the colour-coded bags.

Soiled linen should be placed into the appropriate designated white or clear plastic bag. *Infected linen* is firstly placed into a *water-soluble bag* and then a red outer laundry bag. Other coloured bags for fabrics unable to withstand high water temperatures are also available. Dirty laundry should be stored safely while awaiting transportation to the laundry. Linen is decontaminated through the mechanical process of laundering with detergent and a high water temperature (Arrowsmith 2005). Any microorganisms that are present on the linen, following washing, can be destroyed by ironing and tumble-drying (Wilson 2001).

Spillages of blood or body fluids

All blood/body fluids spillages should be treated as potential biohazards (Pratt *et al.* 2007) and should be dealt with promptly, that is at the time at which they occur. Before dealing with any spillage it is of paramount importance to protect yourself by using PPE. Prior to cleaning, most spillages are disinfected using a high chlorine content releasing agent (sodium hypochlorite). Chlorine-releasing agents *MUST NOT* be used for *urine* spillages as they can react with the fluid and produce chlorine gas.

Sodium hypochlorite is available in many forms and depending upon the type of body fluid different concentrations of sodium hypochlorite may be required. Each organisation will have a spillage policy and it must be recognised that not all spillages will be managed exactly the same in clinical areas. For example, it would be wholly unacceptable to clean up a blood spillage, using sodium hypochlorite, on a carpet within a patient's own home.

Granules have a long shelf life, contain the spillage and require no dilution. The spill should be covered for the manufacturer's recommended time and then mopped up using paper towels.

Tablets – Different brands have different concentrations of product per tablet. The correct number of tablets should be used in the *specified* amount of water to make up a solution of the desired concentration. Follow manufacturer's recommendations to ensure correct dilution. Incorrect dilution could render the disinfectant ineffective.

After clearing the spillage, the area should be cleaned with hot soap and water.

Infection Control and Health Promotion

As a nurse you have a responsibility to maintain your knowledge and clinical skills (NMC 2008). In today's health care provision, education and training sessions are provided by universities, colleges and by health care organisations. These can be formal and informal activities which seek to reinforce existing knowledge and will provide any new evidence that impacts upon any change in practice. You will also learn from your mentor. If there are many students on clinical placement, in a particular health care setting, it may be advantageous to ask if the specialist infection control team could provide a bespoke training/education session for you.

It is not just about education of HCWs but there is also a need to educate patients and their visitors about infection control practices. At the time of writing, there are many local and national campaigns to encourage patients and the public to wash their hands when in hospitals. Do you encourage this activity? Similarly what do you do when you see another HCW omit an infection control activity like hand decontamination? This is where your knowledge of health promotion can be utilised. Consider what health promotion strategy you would employ in maintaining good levels of patient and visitor hand hygiene (Activity 10.7).

Section 3

Activity 10.7

In your clinical placement area, consider a case study or a scenario where there were infection control issues. Using a model of reflection, critically examine the infection control issues that are highlighted. What was your role and that of specialist infection control practitioners in the management of the patient or the situation? Provide a rationale for any recommendations for clinical practice supported by contemporary available evidence. Discuss these issues with your mentor.

Conclusion

Infection control encompasses every area of health care provision and all HCWs are responsible for ensuring safe working practices. Infections are invisible to the naked eye and maintaining patients, in a microbiologically safe environment, is an ever-increasing challenge. You must constantly risk assess all your professional activities and adopt the standard principles for infection control practice with all patients and procedures. You must also comply with employers' policies, protocols and procedures. This will ensure equitable, standardised care practices and minimise the transmission of infection. Failure to comply with policy and best evidence-based practice can result in disciplinary action.

Areas of specialist practice will have more complex skills and knowledge around infection control issues and you will learn about and experience these when working in these areas of practice. However, if you have a clear understanding of the standard principles for infection control, they provide mechanisms to standardise practice, safeguard staff, patients and the organisation. These standard principles also equip you with transferable knowledge and skills into all clinical practice arenas.

The research-based evidence to guide practice may change over time, and you have a responsibility to maintain your knowledge and adapt care practices and skills that reflect that evidence.

Knowledge around infection control practices from laundry management to isolation techniques will enable you to make informed decisions in providing a high standard of patient care when controlling or preventing the spread of infection. This evidence-based knowledge can be utilised in health promotion activities with patients, visitors and other members of staff to change behaviours that reinforce the need for a high standard of infection control practice.

Over time, your acquired knowledge, in tandem with further education, will enable you to further develop in your career pathway to a more specialised level of professional practice. Areas of specialist practice will possibly require more complex and diverse skills and knowledge around infection control issues, but the standard principles for infection control practice can be consolidated and strengthened with a firm researched-evidence base, thus ensuring that you operate, safely, efficiently and maintain a high level of professional practice throughout your professional career (Activity 10.8).

Activity 10.8

Further reading and resources

In order to apply the evidence base for good practice into your day-to-day activities you also need to engage in education and training and study activities around the subject area. However, it is also imperative to have an insight into the social and political drivers for good practice. You should familiarise yourself with the contents of the following key texts and documents.

Key texts

Ayliffe G.A.J., Fraise A.P., Geddes A.M., Mitchell K. (eds) (2000) *Control of Hospital Infection – A Practical Handbook*, 4th edn. Arnold, London.

Bennett P., Calman K. (2001) *Risk Communication and Public Health.* Oxford University Press, Oxford.

Healey J., Spencer M. (2008) *Surviving Your Placement in Health and Social Care: A Student Handbook.* McGraw-Hill, Maidenhead.

Horton R., Parker L. (2002) *Informed Infection Control Practice*, 2nd edn. Churchill Livingstone, London (Chapters 2 and 11 are referred to in the chapter).

Lawrence J., May D. (eds) (2003) *Infection Control in the Community.* Churchill Livingstone, London.

Wilson J. (2001) *Infection Control in Clinical Practice*, 2nd edn. Balliere Tindall, Edinburgh.

Key documents

Department of Health (DH) (2006) *The Health Act 2006: Code of Practice for the Prevention and Control of Healthcare Associated Infections.* Department of Health, London (revised January 2008).

The CDC in Atlanta (2007) recently published new comprehensive guidelines for isolation. http://www.dh.gov.uk/en/Publicationsandstatistics/Publications/PublicationsPolicyAndGuidance/DH_081927

Department of Health (DH) (2006) *Environment and Sustainability.* Health Technical Memorandum 07–01: Safe Management of Healthcare Waste. Department of Health, London.

National Institute for Clinical Excellence (NICE) (2003) *Infection Control Prevention of Healthcare Associated Infection in Primary and Community Care.* National Institute For Clinical Excellence, London.

Pratt R. *et al.* (2007) *Epic2:* National evidence-based guidelines for preventing health care associated infections in NHS hospitals in England. *Journal of Hospital Infection* 65 (Supplement 1).

Section 3

References

Arrowsmith V. (2005) Preventing cross infection. In: *Developing Practical Nursing Skills*, 2nd edn. (ed. Baillie L.). Arnold, London, p. 81.

Ayliffe G.A.J., Fraise A.P., Geddes A.M., Mitchell K. (eds) (2000) *Control of Hospital Infection: A Practical Handbook*, 4th edn. Arnold, London.

Bennett P., Calman K. (2001) *Risk Communication and Public Health*. Oxford University Press, Oxford.

Centre for Disease Control (CDC) (2007) *Standard Precautions* (online), available at http://www.cdc.gov/ncidod/dhqp/gl_isolation_standard.html (accessed 4 February 2008).

Cochrane J. (2000) Moral precepts of handwashing in community practice. *Journal of Community Nursing* 14(10): 19–20.

Cochrane J. (2003) Infection control audit of hand hygiene facilities. *Nursing Standard* 17(18): 33–38.

Dancer S.J. (1999) Mopping up hospital infection. *Journal of Hospital Infection* 43: 85–100.

Denton M., Wilcox M., Parnel P., Green D., Keer V., Hawkey P.M., Evans I. Murphy P. (2004) Role of environmental cleaning in controlling an outbreak of *Acinetobacter baumannii* on a neurosurgical unit. *Journal of Hospital Infection* 56: 106–110.

Department of Health (DH) (2004) *Towards Cleaner Hospitals and Lower Rates of Infection.* Department of Health, London.

Department of Health (DH) (2006a) *The Health Act 2006: Code of Practice for the Prevention and Control of Healthcare Associated Infections.* Department of Health, London (revised January 2008) (online), available at http://www.dh.gov.uk/en/Publicationsandstatistics/Publications/PublicationsPolicyAndGuidance/DH_081927 (accessed 22 January 2008).

Department of Health (DH) (2006b) *Essential Steps to Safe Clean Care.* Department of Health, London.

Department of Health (DH) (2006c) *Environment and Sustainability.* Health Technical Memorandum 07-01: Safe Management of Healthcare Waste. Department of Health, London.

Department of Health (DH) (2007) *Uniforms and Workwear: An Evidence Base for Developing Local Policy.* Department of Health, London.

Hart S. (2007) Using and aseptic to reduce the risk of infection. *Nursing Standard* 21(47): 43–48.

Healey J., Spencer M. (2008) *Surviving Your Placement in Health and Social Care: A Student Handbook.* McGraw-Hill, Maidenhead.

Health and Safety at Work Act (1974) HMSO, London.

Health and Safety Commission (2002) *Control of Substances Hazardous to Health Regulations Approved Codes of Practice.* HSE, London.

Holland S. (2007) *Public Health Ethics.* Polity, Cambridge.

Horton R., Parker L. (2002) *Informed Infection Control Practice,* 2nd edn. Churchill Livingstone, London, Chapter 2.

Keyworth N. (2000) Introduction to microbiology and virology. In: *Infection Control, Science, Management and Practice* (ed. McCulloch J.). Whurr, London, Chapter 2, p. 19.

Lawrence J., May D. (eds) (2003) *Infection Control in the Community.* Churchill Livingstone, London.

McNeill W.H. (1976) *People and Plagues.* Doubleday, New York.

National Health Service Executive (NHSE) (1995) *Hospital Laundry Arrangements for Used and Infected Linen, HSG* (95)18. NHSE, Leeds.

National Institute for Clinical Excellence (NICE) (2003) *Infection Control Prevention of Healthcare Associated Infection in Primary and Community Care.* National Institute for Clinical Excellence, London.

National Patient Safety Agency (NPSA) (2006) *Root Cause Analysis Tool Kit* (online), available at http://www.npsa.nhs.uk/patientsafety/improvingpatientsafety/rootcauseanalysis/

Nursing and Midwifery Council (NMC) (2007) *Essential Skills Clusters.* NMC Circular 07(2007) Annexe 2, NMC, London.

Nursing and Midwifery Council (NMC) (2008) The *Code: Standards of Conduct, Performance and Ethics for Nurses and Midwives.* Nursing and Midwifery Council, London.

Orme J., Powell J., Taylor P., Harrison T., Grey M. (2003) *Public Health for the 21st Century: New Perspectives on Policy, Participation and Practice.* Open University Press, Maidenhead.

Pratt R., Pellowe, C.M., Loveday H.P., Robinson N., Smith G.W. and the epic guideline development team: Barrett S., Davey P., Harper P., Loveday C., McDougall C., Mulhall A., Privett S., Smales C., Taylor L., Weller B., Wilcox M. (2001) Epic Project: developing National evidence-based guidelines for preventing health care associated infections. Phase 1. *Journal of Hospital Infection* 47 (Supplement): S3–S4.

Pratt R., Pellowe C.M., Wilson J.A., Loveday H.P., Harper P.J., Jones S.R.L.J., McDougall C., Wilcox M.H. (2007) *Epic2:* National evidence-based guidelines for preventing health care associated infections in NHS hospitals in England. *Journal of Hospital Infection* 65 (Supplement 1): S1–S59.

Rogers R. (1985) Attitude change and integration in fear appeals. *Psychological Reports* 56: 179–182.

Royal College of Nursing (RCN) (2007) *Safe Management of Health Care Waste*. Royal College of Nursing, London.

Thistlethwaite J., Tie R.N. (2007) Learning and teaching about risk communication. *The Clinical Teacher* 4: 135–140.

Wilson J. (2001) *Infection Control in Clinical Practice*, 2nd edn. Ballière Tindall, London, p. 75.

Section 4

Nutrition and Fluid Management

Section 4

CHAPTER 11

Principles of Nutrition

Sue M. Green

Introduction

The NMC Essential Skills Clusters (NMC 2007) for pre-registration nursing programmes outlines the skills required for nurses in relation to patient nutrition. This chapter briefly outlines nutritional concepts that are relevant to care of patients/clients and considers the role of the nurse in nutritional care.

The specific learning outcomes addressed in this chapter link with the Nursing and Midwifery Council's (NMC 2007) Essential Skills Clusters, and are identified below.

Learning outcomes

By the end of this chapter you will be able to do the following:

- Discuss critically how the nurse can provide assistance with selecting a diet through which patients/clients will receive adequate nutritional and fluid intake.
- Describe comprehensively how the nurse can assess and monitor nutritional status and formulate an effective care plan.
- Identify how to provide an environment conducive to eating and drinking.
- Review how the nurse can ensure that those unable to take food by mouth receive adequate nutrition.

Nurses are required to be able to use their "*knowledge of dietary and other factors contributing to ill health, obesity, weight loss, poor fluid intake and poor nutrition to inform practice*" (NMC 2007, p. 21). It is important, therefore, to have an understanding of the principles of nutritional science and the effects of poor nutritional intake on health.

Nutrients and Factors which may Influence Nutritional Intake

The body needs nutrients to enable cells to carry out the processes needed to sustain life. Nutrients are used

- to provide energy for metabolic processes that support physical activity, growth, pregnancy and lactation;
- to produce structural materials; and
- to form parts of the enzymic processes which take place in the body.

Nutrients are categorised as macronutrients and micronutrients. Macronutrients include protein, fat and carbohydrate, and provide the body with energy and structural substances to enable growth and repair. Micronutrients are vitamins and minerals. These form structural components of the body and are a part of many of the biochemical processes in the body. Alcohol can be considered to be a macronutrient in that it is metabolised by the body to produce energy. It is, however, not an essential nutrient and excessive intakes are toxic.

Protein

The smallest unit of a protein is an amino acid. A number of amino acids joined together form a protein. There are about 20 amino acids that are important for a patient's/client's health. Some of these can be manufactured in the body (termed non-essential amino acids) and some have to be consumed as they cannot be made in the body (termed essential amino acids). Protein forms many components of the body, for example muscle, hormones and skin and is required for growth and repair of tissues. Rich protein sources include soya, nuts, cheese and meat. A lack of protein leads to muscle wastage; however, a very high intake can be detrimental to health (AHA 2008).

Fat

The main types of fats used by the body are triglycerides and cholesterol. Triglycerides consist of glycerol and fatty acids, which may be saturated, monounsaturated, polyunsaturated or trans-saturated. The term saturation refers to the chemical structure of the fatty acid. Two types of polyunsaturated fatty acids, linoleic acid and a-linolenic acid, are termed essential fatty acids. Cholesterol is a type of fat that is present in animal tissues as a component of cell membranes and also forms bile acids and some hormones. The body makes its own cholesterol and, therefore, a dietary source is not essential. Fat is transported in the blood stream within lipoproteins, which have been implicated in the development of heart disease. Fat is an important nutrient and is used by the body to produce energy and to provide insulation and protection. Fat is also needed to make cell membranes and some hormones.

Saturated fats are generally solid at room temperature. Unsaturated fats tend to be liquid at room temperature. Most foods contain a mix of the different types of fatty acids but are rich in one type. Rich sources of saturated fats include animal products such as butter and red meat. Rich sources of monounsaturated fat include some plant oils, such as olive oil and some nuts and seeds. Polyunsaturated fats are present in large amounts in oily fish and plant oils such as sunflower oil. Trans-saturated fatty acids are found in large amounts in processed products such as biscuits.

For optimal health a moderate fat intake, which includes an adequate amount of essential fatty acids and a low intake of saturated fats, should be consumed. Lack of dietary fat intake is detrimental to health and can lead to an inadequate intake of the fat-soluble vitamins such as vitamin D.

Carbohydrate

The smallest unit of a carbohydrate is a monosaccharide. There are three main types of monosaccharide used by the body: glucose, fructose and galactose. Two monosaccharides joined together form a disaccharide (such as sucrose and lactose). Many monosaccharide units joined together form a polysaccharide. Polysaccharides which are important to human nutrition include starch and non-starch polysaccharides. Non-starch polysaccharides (NSP) are not digested by enzymes produced by the gastrointestinal (GI) tract and are more commonly known as fibre.

Carbohydrate is used by the body to provide energy for cells. If carbohydrate is not available for body cells to use then body stores of fat and protein will be used to provide energy for the cells. NSP is required for the GI tract to function properly and move food components through at an appropriate rate. Carbohydrate intake should mostly take the form of complex carbohydrates (i.e. starch and NSP). Intake of sucrose and fructose, often called 'simple sugars', that has been refined from plant sources should be limited. Rich sources of complex carbohydrates include vegetables, fruits, grains and pulses.

Micronutrients

Vitamins known to promote nutritional health include A, thiamine (B_1), riboflavin (B_2), niacin (B_3), pyridoxine (B_6), B_{12}, biotin, pantothenic acid, C, D, E, K and folate. Minerals known to be essential for health include calcium, phosphorous, magnesium, sodium, potassium, chloride, iron, zinc, copper, selenium and iodine. Other micronutrients are also required by the body in small amounts.

Generally speaking, a healthy patient/client can derive all the micronutrients he or she requires from eating a diet containing all the major food groups in appropriate amounts. However, some groups in the United Kingdom may commonly experience a deficiency of micronutrients such as iron, folate, calcium and B_{12}. For example people who drink large amounts of alcohol may be deficient in thiamine and other B vitamins. A patient/client who is unwell or is receiving medical treatment may benefit from micronutrient supplementation as he or she may not be eating properly or his or her condition or treatment may affect absorption and utilisation of nutrients. The very unwell patient/client will usually require close monitoring of the level of micronutrients which act to help to maintain homeostasis, for example potassium and sodium.

Taking amounts of nutrients in excess of the recommended amount can lead to poor health (Food Standards Agency (FSA) 2003).

Section 4

A healthy diet

A patient's/client's 'diet' consists of the foods he or she eats from day to day. A diet that contains all the nutrients the body requires, in the appropriate amounts, is essential for good health. The student nurse should have an understanding of the nutritional requirements of a healthy patient/client on entry to branch (NMC 2007). Information on the nutritional requirements for healthy people can be seen on the FSA website (FSA 2008). Calculating the nutritional requirements of a patient/client who is unwell is complex and usually undertaken by the dietitian in the clinical setting.

The recommended diet for a healthy patient/client is shown in Figure 11.1 using the health promotion tool termed the 'eatwell plate'.

This type of diet is considered to promote the health of the people living in the United Kingdom best. The tips for eating well issued by the FSA (2008) are shown in Box 11.1. Eating a wide variety of foods promotes health as it is easier to obtain all the nutrients essential for a healthy diet.

Not all people are able to follow the type of diet described in the *Eatwell Plate*. Some may eat a therapeutic diet prescribed by the dietitian, such as a gluten-free diet and some may need to eat modified foods such as pureed foods. A small number of people may not consume all their nutrient needs orally but have an infusion of nutrients into the stomach or small bowel by tube (enteral nutrition) or directly into the blood stream (parenteral nutrition (PN)).

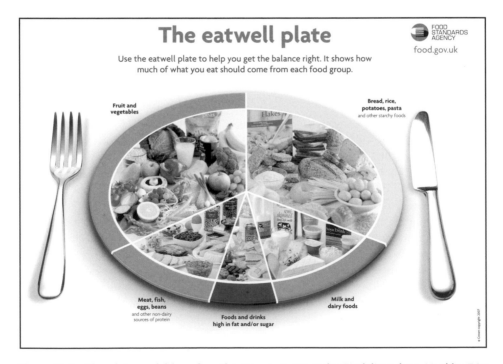

Figure 11.1   The plate model based on the Government's Eight Guidelines for a Healthy Diet (FSA 2007). © Crown copyright material is reproduced with the permission of the Controller of HMSO and Queen's Printer for Scotland.

> **BOX 11.1**
>
> **Eight tips for eating well (FSA 2008)**
>
> 1. Base your meals on starchy foods
> 2. Eat lots of fruits and vegetables
> 3. Eat more fish
> 4. Cut down on saturated fat and sugar
> 5. Try to eat less salt – no more than 6 g a day
> 6. Get active and try to be a healthy weight
> 7. Drink plenty of water
> 8. Do not skip breakfast.

Factors affecting food intake

All nurses working with patients/clients to enable them to change their diet need to understand what factors may influence food intake.

The type of diet a patient/client chooses to consume is influenced by their socio-economic situation. If foods are not available to buy or cannot be grown then they will not be consumed. This is the over-riding factor in food choice in areas where there are food shortages. Where foods stuffs are available to buy, a patient/client must be able to access where they are sold, have the money to buy them and the means to transport them home. At home, in order to store and prepare food, storage and cooking facilities are required. If the process of food acquisition and preparation is limited the quality of the diet may be affected.

If a wide variety of food is available and can be readily acquired and prepared, the amount and type of food a patient/client chooses to eat will depend on a number of factors including culture, appetite, psychological factors and health.

Cultural issues influence the type of foods that a patient/client eats and, therefore, it is important for the nurse to ascertain patients'/clients' dietary preferences to ensure that they are offered foods that are culturally acceptable to them.

A patient's/client's *appetite* will influence dietary intake. The body regulates how much is eaten by various physiological and psychological mechanisms. Physiological mechanisms include the stomach emptying and filling, the presence of nutrients in the small intestine, levels of gastro-intestinal (GI) hormones and glucose levels in the blood. External cues are also important, for example, the smell of food helps to prepare the body physiologically for food ingestion. External cues can also act to reduce food intake. This is particularly important in acute units where noxious smells and sights, such as someone vomiting nearby, can reduce a patient's appetite.

Psychological factors are also important. People diagnosed with anorexia nervosa or bulimia have a disordered response to their hunger drive and will eat far too little or too much to meet their nutritional needs. Mental states, such as confusion, distress and depression, can influence food choice and the amount of food eaten. For example, people diagnosed with dementia may go through a period of hyperphagia when they eat large amounts of food and a period of diminished appetite.

Some medical conditions will influence dietary intake. Medical conditions that cause dysphagia, such as stroke, may lead to a patient/client being unable to eat anything orally being prescribed a textured modified diet so that swallowing is facilitated. There are a number of medical conditions that affect the way some foods are digested in the GI tract. For example, a patient/client with coeliac's disease cannot digest gluten (present in wheat) and, therefore, must avoid wheat-based products. People with inflammatory bowel disease may find avoiding some foods helpful in managing their symptoms, and people with a colostomy or illeostomy are advised to avoid certain foods to help them to manage flatus, diarrhoea or constipation. In hospital settings, patients may be made 'nil by mouth' for extended periods of time as part of preparation for theatre or investigations reducing nutritional intake. Patients who have had bowel surgery are usually ordered not to eat after surgery until the surgeon is satisfied that the bowel is functioning properly.

The way food is metabolised in the body may affect the type of foods eaten. Some people are unable to metabolise certain components of food due to a genetic disorder. The best known example of this is phenylketonuria, which is a genetic error in metabolism of the amino acid phenylalanine. All newborns in the United Kingdom are screened for this disorder as avoidance of phenylalanine from birth is important to enable normal development.

Medical treatments for some conditions may cause symptoms that affect food intake and food choice. For example, chemotherapy often causes nausea. Some medications interact with components of food, this is termed a 'drug–nutrient interaction'. An example of this is the interaction between monoamine oxidase inhibitors (which are sometimes prescribed for depression) and tyramine (an amino acid) metabolism which can result in a hypertensive crisis. Therefore, foods high in tyramine such as cheese, processed meats, broad beans and soya need to be avoided. The pharmacist will usually review each patient's/client's prescribed medications and highlight the potential for any drug–nutrient interaction by providing appropriate instructions for the administration of the medications. The nurse needs to be aware of common drug–nutrient interactions and ensure that the patient/client is well informed of how to avoid potential problems.

Malnutrition and the effects of poor nutrition

Malnutrition may refer to both excessive nutritional intake (over-nutrition) and inadequate nutritional intake (under-nutrition). Generally speaking, in the United Kingdom, when the term malnutrition is used it refers to an inadequate intake, most commonly a low intake of protein and energy (or kilocalories). Some people do have other nutrient deficiencies such as iron deficiency anaemia. Those at risk of malnutrition include those of a low socio-economic status, older adults, and those living in institutions (Brownie 2006). However, it is important to be aware that increasingly over-nutrition is affecting health. Obesity is a major global public health issue and nurses are becoming more involved in the management of obesity.

Poor nutritional intake can have far-reaching effects. Excessive as well as insufficient nutrients can compromise how the body functions. A high intake of energy can lead to obesity, which increases the risk of the development of cardiovascular

---

Activity 11.1

Further reading and resources

British Association for Parenteral & Enteral Nutrition (2008) *Welcome to BAPEN*, available at http://www.bapen.org.uk/ (accessed 1 April 2008).

DoH (2003) *The Essence of Care: Patient-focused Benchmarks for Clinical Governance.* HMSO, London.

Food Standards Agency (2008) *Nutrition,* available at http://www.food.gov.uk/healthiereating/ (accessed 31 March 2008).

Mental Health Foundation (2008) *Food & Mental Health Campaign*, available at http://www.mentalhealth.org.uk/campaigns/food-and-mental-health/ (accessed 4 January 2008).

National Collaborating Centre for Acute Care (2006) *Nutrition Support in Adults: Oral Nutrition Support, Enteral Tube Feeding and Parenteral Nutrition.* National Collaborating Centre for Acute Care, London, available at http://www.nice.org.uk/page.aspx?o=cg032 (accessed.1 December 2008).

Royal College of Nursing (RCN) (2006) *Malnutrition. What Nurses Working with Children and Young People Need to Know and Do.* RCN, London.

---

disease and Type-II diabetes mellitus as well as some other conditions. A high intake of saturated fats can increase the risk of developing atherosclerosis. At the other end of the spectrum, a reduced dietary intake can lead to weight loss and the development of disorders associated with specific nutrient deficiencies such as anaemia and rickets. Undernourished patients in hospital are more likely to spend longer in hospital and develop conditions such as pressure ulcers and chest infections as they have less resource with which to mobilise, fight infection, repair tissue and build new tissue.

The second part of this chapter focuses on the nutritional care of people by nurses. Activity 11.1 provides further reading on this topic.

Assessing and Monitoring Nutritional Status and Formulating an Effective Care Plan

Nursing care is a systematic process and *nutritional care* should be considered in the same way. Figure 11.2 shows the process of nutritional care. The first part of the process involves screening patients/clients to identify those at risk of malnutrition and those with particular dietary requirements. Those who are considered to be at risk of malnutrition should then be assessed fully to identify the issues of concern and referred to other members of the multidisciplinary team (MDT) as appropriate. If patients/clients have particular dietary requirements, a full assessment of their particular needs must take place. Following assessment a plan of care should be devised, implemented and then evaluated to ensure that nutritional needs are meet. Each stage of this process is discussed below.

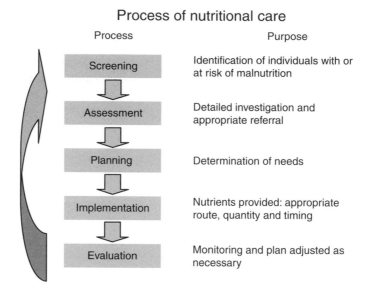

Figure 11.2   The process of nutritional care (adapted from McLaren & Green 1998).

Screening and Assessment

In order to provide good nutritional care to a patient/client the nurse must first screen for potential or actual problems. If a problem is identified then nutritional status and the factors influencing it can be assessed thoroughly.

The nurse should be able to make 'a comprehensive assessment of patients'/clients' needs in relation to nutrition identifying, documenting and communicating level of risk' (NMC 2007, p. 22). The NMC (2007, p. 22) highlights that the student nurse on entry to branch should be able to take and record 'accurate measurements of weight, height, length, Body Mass Index (BMI) and other appropriate measures of nutritional status'. There are several ways in which a nurse can screen for malnutrition and assess nutritional status.

Nutritional screening tools

It is recommended that all adult patients/clients are screened for malnutrition using a simple nutritional screening tool (NICE 2006). Nutritional screening tools are a quick and easy way to screen for malnutrition and document a patient's/client's nutritional status. There are numerous tools available, but it is important to ensure that any tool used has been shown to be valid and reliable (Green & Watson 2005). One widely used screening tool that has been shown to be valid and reliable is the Malnutrition Universal Screening Tool (BAPEN 2006).

Assessment of body composition

The simplest assessment of body composition is weight and height from which BMI can be calculated. BMI allows consideration of weight in relation to height and gives a simple indication as to whether a patient/client is underweight, normal weight, overweight or obese. However, BMI must be used in conjunction with clinical judgement as patients/clients with high muscle mass, for example contact sports players, usually have a high BMI which may suggest they are overweight when in fact they actually have a low fat mass. Giving dietary advice based on a BMI to an older patient/client also needs to be considered very carefully. There is some evidence to suggest that an older patient/client with a BMI of over 26 may be able to recover from illness better than one with a lower BMI and, therefore, losing weight is not advisable (British Dietetics Association 2003).

In primary care, waist circumference can be used to screen for cardiovascular risk, as it can give a quick indication of the amount of abdominal fat. A waist circumference of greater than 102 cm in men and 88 cm in women indicates that advice on how weight can be reduced may be beneficial (Lean 2000). However, as with BMI, this measure may not be appropriate for use with older adults, particularly the very old.

Other methods of assessment of body composition, including bio-impedance analysis and skin-fold thickness measurement, can be used by nurses but additional training is required to ensure competency in undertaking the measurement.

Laboratory assessment

Measurement of nutrients in blood and other tissues can give an indication of nutritional status, although the level may be influenced by disease state rather than nutritional status. For example, serum protein values may indicate malnutrition, but can also be affected by factors other than nutritional status such as liver disease. As the interpretation of laboratory assessments with respect to nutritional status is complex, the results of any tests need to be considered by the MDT.

Dietary history

It is important to assess patients'/clients' usual dietary intake and any factors influencing the quantity and types of foods eaten. Information can be obtained by asking the patients/clients, their carers or relatives or reading the patients' nursing and medical records. The NMC (2007, p. 22) highlights that the student nurse at entry to branch should be able to contribute 'to formulating a care plan through assessment of dietary preferences, including local availability of foods and cooking facilities'.

Assessment of dietary intake

Current or recent dietary intake can be assessed simply by the use of a food chart, asking the patient/client to recall food eaten in the previous 24 hours or recording of a food diary.

A food chart is used when dietary intake of a patient/client in a care setting needs to be monitored in order to assess the adequacy of nutritional intake. Completion of a food chart involves the accurate recording of foods and nutritious fluids consumed. It is important that a food chart is completed with the highest degree of accuracy possible and that the intake is added up and related to the patient's/client's needs and appropriate action taken.

Section 4

Activity 11.2

Discuss with your mentor how patients/clients are nutritionally screened and assessed in your area of practice.

Memory recall of dietary intake over the previous 24 hours involves asking the patient/client to recall exactly what they have eaten over the previous day. This is a useful method of dietary assessment if a patient/client is admitted with an illness which is suspected to be related to recent food intake.

When the nurse is facilitating a patient to change their dietary habits, asking them to keep a food diary over the course of 7 days can be useful. This will enable the nurse to work with the patient/client to determine aspects of the diet that the patient/client can change, for example, grilling food instead of frying it or reducing the number of snacks eaten.

These methods of screening and assessment are also used to evaluate care, which is discussed later in the chapter (Activity 11.2).

Planning Care

Nurses should take 'action to ensure that, where there are problems with eating and swallowing, nutritional status is not compromised' (NMC 2007, p. 23). Following screening and assessment, a plan of care needs to be formulated to outline the actions to be taken to address the problems identified. The plan of care may form part of a care pathway or care plan. The patient/client should be involved in the care planning process where possible. Nurses are required to provide information to patients/clients and carers (NMC 2007) and develop the plan of care with the patient/client where possible.

Nurses are expected to seek 'specialist advice as required in order to formulate an appropriate care plan' (NMC 2007, p. 22). If a patient or client is found to be at risk of malnutrition, be it under- or over-malnutrition or a poor dietary intake, referral to another member of the MDT may be appropriate. This will usually not only include the dietitian and the doctor but may also include others such as the speech and language therapist (SALT) or the occupational therapist. If the patient/client has been referred to another member of the MDT, their plan of action for the patient/client must be detailed in the care plan.

Implementing Care

Once a care plan has been formulated it needs to be implemented. If aspects of the care plan cannot be implemented by the nurse caring for the patient/client, the nurse should refer to other members of the MDT for additional or specialist advice (NMC 2007). Many Trusts have a Nutrition Support Team (NST) to which patients/clients can be referred to if required. An NST provides specialist advice concerning nutritional support and usually consists not only of a doctor, nurse specialist, dietitian and pharmacist but may also include others such as a biochemist.

Promoting healthy eating

The nurse is required to support 'patients/clients to make appropriate choices/changes to eating patterns, taking account of dietary preferences (including religious and cultural requirements) and "therapeutic" diets needed for health reasons' (NMC 2007, p. 21). This involves discussion with patients/clients about 'how diet can improve health and the risks associated with not eating appropriately' (NMC 2007, p. 21). Student nurses on entry to branch should be able to support patients/clients to make healthy food and fluid choices under supervision (NMC 2007). Facilitating dietary change should be done by using appropriate health promotion strategies. Food consumption is a behaviour, and in order to change behaviour the factors influencing the behaviour need to be explored with the patient/client in order to consider how to change the behaviour. It is important that any advice given is culturally appropriate. If a patient/client has been prescribed a therapeutic diet by the dietitian any advice given by the nurse must be consistent with that given by the dietitian. Nurses working with children should be able to provide 'advice and support to mothers who are breastfeeding' (NMC 2007, p. 21).

Patients/clients should generally be encouraged to adhere to the UK healthy eating guidelines (FSA 2008). However, it is important to remember that people who are under-malnourished or at risk of under-malnourishment need a high-energy diet and need to be offered foods that they find appetising. Therefore, they should not restrict their intake of energy, high fat and high sugar foods.

Providing an environment conducive to eating and drinking (NMC 2007)

It is important that the nurse ensures that the environment a patient/client eats in encourages him or her to eat and drink by considering the mealtime surroundings and activities that take place at that time, and ensuring food and drinks are available as required. This issue particularly concerns residential care settings but may involve considering the home environment if necessary.

The nurse should ensure that appropriate food and fluids are available as required (NMC 2007) and dietary preferences are met. The recent *Hungry to be Heard* report (Age Concern 2006) suggested that despite labels attached to each menu, patients and clients were given inappropriate food at times. Clearly, it is important that all staff adhere to the patient's/client's plan of care and that volunteers involved in any aspect of nutritional care and the patient's/client's visitors must also be fully aware of any particular dietary needs. Relatives and carers can bring in favourite foods if local policy allows and can assist the patient/client to eat and drink where appropriate.

The student nurse should be able to explain the rationale for a particular type of diet prescribed and support the patient/client who needs to adhere to specific dietary and fluid regimes (NMC 2007). Patients/clients are sometimes required to follow a restrictive diet that is very difficult for them to adhere to, so it is important that they are supported appropriately. Patients/clients who have undergone surgery will normally be advised by the surgeon as to when they may start eating

Section 4

and drinking and what types of food and drink they may eat over the course of the recovery period. Patients/clients should be nil by mouth for only as long as is indicated medically and given food or drink promptly as soon as they may eat or drink.

Activities should be limited at mealtimes to enable nutritional care to be the focus of care at those times. The concept of 'Protected Mealtimes' has been introduced recently in some hospitals (Davidson & Scholefield 2005) to try to limit interruptions at mealtimes and some clinical areas use a 'red tray system' whereby patients/clients are served their food on a red tray if they require assistance at mealtimes (Age Concern 2006). The student nurse should be aware of and follow local procedures in relation to mealtimes (NMC 2007). Unpleasant sounds, sights and smells can affect appetite. Steps should be taken to try to avoid factors which discourage eating, for example, offering toileting facilities before mealtimes.

Food safety is an important issue in health care settings and it is important that everyone involved in food-related activities, including the student nurse, follows food hygiene procedures (NMC 2007).

The student nurse should report to his or her mentor or an appropriate nurse if a patient/client is unable to eat at a mealtime as the nurse should make 'provision for replacement meals for those ... unable to eat at the usual time' (NMC 2007, p. 23). Food and drinks should be available over the 24-hour period, so a patient/client who has missed a meal can still eat sufficiently to meet their nutritional needs. Many care settings have the facility of a 24-hour menu. If this is not available then replacement meal products (e.g. soup) and nutritional supplements should be available in the unit kitchen. A patient/client may also have food products stored in his or her bedside cabinet which relatives have brought in.

Oral nutritional food supplements may be prescribed if a patient/client requires his or her diet to be supplemented. These take the form of drinks, soups or puddings. Depending on the clinical setting they may be prescribed by the dietitian or doctor, or nurses may be able to use them as necessary. The palatability and presentation of the supplement should be considered carefully. The drinks often taste better served cold, although some flavours may taste pleasant gently warmed for example chocolate. The drinks can be mixed with other foods and drinks if this enhances the palatability, for example vanilla flavour may replace milk served with breakfast cereal.

Providing assistance at mealtimes

This involves a wide range of activities including assisting the patient/client to choose a meal from a hospital menu. The NMC (2007) highlights that the student nurse at entry to branch should be able to provide assistance as required and that the nurse should ensure that 'appropriate assistance and support is available to enable patients/clients to eat' (NMC 2007, p. 23).

In a recent report entitled *Hungry to be Heard* (Age Concern 2006), nine out of ten nurses suggested that they did not always have time to help ensure hospital patients eat properly. The report suggested that some patients were not given appropriate assistance to eat, for example, meals arrived with the cover on and were taken away with the cover still on and relatives of patients were forced to start a rota to ensure that everyone was assisted to eat. The NMC Code (NMC 2008) states that the nurse must protect and support the health of individual patients and clients. Nurses are, therefore, responsible for ensuring that a patient/client receives appropriate nutritional care.

The student nurse on entry to branch should be able to ensure that patients/ clients are ready for their meal (NMC 2007). Prior to a meal being served, a patient/client should be assisted to use the toilet if required and offered hand washing facilities. Appropriate interventions should be carried out if the patient/client is experiencing pain or nausea. The table the patient/client eats from should be cleaned and clutter removed. In non-acute settings patients/clients should have the facility to be able to eat with others although it should be noted that some prefer to eat by themselves.

Many patients/clients are able to eat and drink independently but require some assistance with mealtime care. Table 11.1 shows the steps that should be taken when providing assistance for a patient/client able to eat and drink. Some patients/clients require assistance to eat and drink as they are unable to do it for themselves. Table 11.2 shows the steps that should be taken when assisting a patient/client to eat and drink.

It is important to stop giving food and fluid to patients/clients and report to the nurse in charge if their voice sounds wet or gurgly, or they show of signs of choking or food is pocketing in their mouth as this suggests food and drink is not

Table 11.1 Providing assistance to the patient/client able to eat and drink independently.

Action	Rationale
• offer facilities to wash hands	• to reduce the risk of microbiological contamination
• ensure positioned correctly (sitting upright unless contraindicated)	• to facilitate ingestion and swallowing and reduce the risk of reflux
• if required ensure feeding aids clean and available	• to reduce the risk of microbiological contamination and to facilitate eating
• if requested by patients/clients provide protection for clothes	• some patients/clients may wish to protect their clothing but some may not
• ensure a drink available if offering food	• to facilitate the swallowing of food
• serve food and drink at the correct temperature	• food served at the correct temperature is more appetising although patients/clients should not be served food or drink with which they can burn themselves
• place food and drink within reach	• many patients/clients can eat independently if food is within reach
• remove covers and prepare food if appropriate	• many patients/clients can eat independently if food is prepared appropriately
• if a patient/client has poor sight describe the food served and indicate where it is placed on the plate using a 'clock face'	• describing food assists the patient/client to prepare to eat their meal
• prompt to eat or drink if needed	• a patient/client with cognitive deficits may become distracted during a meal

Section 4

Table 11.2   Providing assistance for the patients/clients unable to eat and drink unaided.

Procedure	Rationale
• check the patient's/client's dietary needs	• the nurse should ensure that appropriate food and fluids are available as required by a patient/client (NMC 2007)
• introduce yourself, explain the procedure and obtain consent	• informed consent is required from legally competent patients/clients before any care is given (NMC 2008)
• set up the area appropriately	• to reduce the risk of microbiological contamination
• position the patient/client correctly (sitting upright unless contraindicated)	• to facilitate ingestion and swallowing and reduce the risk of reflux
• ensure the patient's/client's mouth is clean and dentures are in place if requested by the patient/client	• to enhance the taste of the food and facilitate chewing and swallowing
• if requested by patient/client provide protection for clothes	• some patients/clients may wish to protect their clothing but some may not
• wash your hands and put on an apron appropriate for serving food	• to reduce the risk of microbiological contamination
• prepare equipment, food and drink needed	• to ensure the procedure is uninterrupted
• sit or stand at the same eye level as the patient/client	• to facilitate communication
• check the food and drink is not too hot before giving it to the patient/client	• patients/clients should not be served food or drink with which they can burn themselves
• give small amounts to the patient/client each mouthful	• to facilitate swallowing
• ensure each mouthful is swallowed	• to avoid food accumulating in the mouth
• pause between offering mouthfuls	• to avoid the patient/client feeling rushed
• offer fluid periodically	• to facilitate swallowing
• communicate with the patient/client to ascertain the pace of feeding is suitable for them and that they are enjoying their meal	• to enhance the patient's/client's experience
• when the patient/client has finished eating offer a mouthwash or check mouth for retained food. If food is retained it can be cleared with a drink, swab or toothbrush	• to promote mouth hygiene
• the patient/client should stay sitting up right for at least 30 minutes (unless contraindicated) to reduce chance of reflux	• to reduce the risk of reflux
• the amount eaten and drunk and any issues of importance should be documented	• to accurately monitor diet and fluid intake and complete relevant documentation (NMC 2007)
	• to report any changes in the patient's/client's condition

being swallowed as it should be. The student nurse should be able to recognise, respond appropriately and report patients/clients who have difficulty in eating or swallowing (NMC 2007).

Patients/clients with swallow deficits may require diet and fluids that are texture modified (e.g. thickened fluids and puree diet). The student nurse should adhere to a plan of care that provides adequate nutrition and hydration when eating or swallowing is difficult (NMC 2007). A texture-modified diet can be unpalatable and it is important that fluids are thickened appropriately and made as pleasant as possible. Support and advice should be provided by nurses to carers when there are feeding difficulties (NMC 2007) as they can support the patient/client and often assist the patient/client to eat and drink where appropriate.

Enteral nutrition by tube and parenteral nutrition (PN)

Nurses should 'ensure that those unable to take food by mouth receive adequate nutrition' (NMC 2007, p. 23). Enteral nutrition by tube is indicated when a patient/client has a functioning GI tract but is unable to eat or swallow sufficient to meet their nutritional needs. PN is indicated when the GI tract is not functioning sufficiently to enable the patient/client to meet his or her nutritional needs. The decision to commence enteral nutrition by tube or PN should be made following discussion with the MDT and where appropriate the patient/client and next of kin.

Enteral nutrition by tube

There are various routes through which the nutrients can be delivered by tube into the GI tract. For short-term feeding a tube which passes through the nose to the stomach (termed a nasoGastric (NG) tube) is used. Less commonly, the tube may pass through the nose to the duodenum (nasoduodenal tube) or jejunum (nasojejunal tube). Very rarely the tube may pass through the mouth into the GI tract. For longer-term feeding a gastrostomy is used. This type of tube passes through the abdominal wall into the stomach and can be inserted radiologically (RIG), percutaneously endoscopically (PEG) or surgically. Rarely the tube may pass through the abdominal wall into the jejunum (jejunumostomy).

NG and gastrostomy tubes are commonly used to provide nutritional support. Therefore, nurses should on entry to the register (where relevant to their branch) be able to safely insert NG tubes and maintain and use NG and gastrostomy tubes (NMC 2007).

The type of tube used is usually determined by local policy. NG tubes can be made of polyvinyl chloride (PVC) or polyurethane. The PVC tubes, often termed 'ryles tubes', are more rigid than polyurethane tubes and need to be changed more frequently. The polyurethane tubes are flexible and, therefore, need a guide wire for insertion. Size 6–8 French Gauge (FG) should be used for feeding purposes.

NG tubes can be inserted by nurses except where patients/clients have maxillo-facial or oesophageal disorders or have undergone maxillofacial surgery or laryngectomy (BAPEN 1996). Local policy and procedure should be consulted prior to the procedure being undertaken. The procedure for insertion of an NG tube is shown in Dougherty and Lister (2008).

Section 4

Following insertion, the position of the NG tube should be checked and documented. The correct way, currently, to ascertain the position of an NG tube is shown on the National Patient Safety Agency website (NPSA 2005). The position should be checked following insertion, before feeding commences, if discomfort or feed reflux into the mouth is experienced and following vomiting, coughing or suctioning. The tube should be secured to the face to avoid displacement.

If it is anticipated that the patient/client will receive enteral feeding by tube for longer than a few weeks the decision to insert a gastrostomy tube may be made by the medical team. A gastrostomy tube may be inserted in theatre, or in the X-ray or Endoscopy Departments. The pre-operative and post-operative care should follow local guidelines. The tract the tube passes through usually takes 2–3 weeks to heal. Once healed the tube should be rotated according to Trust guidelines to prevent tissue adhering to the tube. The position of the tube should be checked daily to ensure it has not changed (indicating displacement of the tube). The site can be cleaned daily with soap and water once healed. Accidental removal of the tube requires prompt action as the tract can close quickly.

Where relevant to their branch nurses on entry to the register should be able to administer enteral feeds safety and maintain the equipment to do this (NMC 2007). Gastrostomy and NG tubes should be flushed regularly to avoid them becoming blocked (BAPEN 1999).

A patient who is critically ill may not digest food properly leading to a build-up of feed in the stomach. For this reason absorption of feed should be checked according to local guidelines.

The type of feed infused and the rate at which it should be given should be prescribed by the dietitian as patients'/clients' nutritional needs can vary. The feed should be given via a volumetric pump to ensure that it is delivered at an appropriate rate. The administration set should be changed as dictated by local guidelines and the pump kept clean to reduce infection risk.

When a patient is receiving a feed, his or her head and shoulders should be elevated by at least 30° during feeding, and, for 1 hour after (unless contraindicated) to avoid reflux into the oesophagus (BAPEN 1999). Medications may be administered via an enteral feed tube provided that they are appropriate for administration via this route. The pharmacist should review the medications prescribed and identify how they should be prepared for administration via the tube.

When a patient/client has an enteral tube *in situ*, their mouth may become dry and less clean as the action of chewing and swallowing stimulates saliva and removes debris in the mouth. Therefore, regular mouth care must be given. It is important that the nurse observes the nasal region carefully if an NG tube is in place as the tube can cause pressure damage on parts of the nose. Pressure damage should be suspected if the patient complains of pain in the nose area or if an area of the nose shows skin changes. The patient/client may also require assistance to clear his or her nose.

Complications associated with enteral tubes include tube displacement, tube blockage and aspiration. Gastrostomy tubes may also be associated with skin excoriation and leakage. Complications associated with enteral feeding by tube include malabsorption of feed, diarrhoea or constipation and biochemical disturbances. It is important, therefore, to closely monitor the patient/client with an

---

Activity 11.3

Locate and read the guidelines on enteral nutrition in your area of practice.

---

enteral tube, observing tube position, clinical condition, fluid balance, temperature, pulse and respiration, weight and bowel habits. Biochemical levels should be monitored by the MDT when enteral feeding by tube is introduced because of the potential problem of refeeding syndrome.

A patient/client may be discharged home with enteral feeding by tube in progress. Discharge planning needs to take place well in advance of the discharge date and involve the MDT in acute and primary care.

Local guidelines concerning the insertion of NG tubes and the care of patient/client with an NG tube should be consulted and further reading on this topic undertaken (Activity 11.3).

Parenteral nutrition

Parenteral nutrition (PN) can be described as the delivery of macronutrients and micronutrients directly into the blood stream. A select or complete range of nutrients may be given. In the United Kingdom, PN is usually administered by the nurse who has undergone additional training in the handling of PN. This is because the risk of infection is high in this type of nutritional support.

It is recommended that an NST should be involved when the decision to give PN is made (BAPEN 1996). This has been suggested to reduce the complications associated with this method of nutritional support.

PN is given via a dedicated line or lumen and is generally given into a central vein although in the short term it can be given peripherally. PN is prescribed by the NST or the Medical Team in association with the pharmacist. It is introduced progressively and the patient is closely monitored as it may cause electrolyte imbalances when it is commenced. Basic monitoring by the ward nursing team involves the measurement of temperature, pulse, respiration, blood glucose level and observation of the catheter entry site. PN is given using a volumetric pump to ensure that the feed is given at the correct rate. PN is an invasive and complex therapy. Complications associated with this type of nutritional support are common and include line-related problems, infection and fluid and electrolyte imbalance.

Psychosocial issues

The impact on normal daily life of drastically changing eating habits should not be underestimated. Eating and drinking is part of our everyday life. It provides structure to our day, enables us to express cultural and religious beliefs and provides a vehicle with which to celebrate events. Removing or reducing the ability to eat and drink normally and giving nutritional support by tube will have a psychological and social (psychosocial) impact on a patient's/client's life and the people with which they share their life.

Activity 11.4

Visit the following website to learn more about how people on this nutritional therapy can be supported: http://www.pinnt.co.uk/index.htm

---

The psychosocial impact will depend on the length of time nutritional support is given and a patient's/client's cognitive ability to appraise the situation. For example, if a patient/client receives a nasogastric feed for 7 days when acutely ill, the psychosocial impact is likely to be much less than a patient/client who is informed that they will require parenteral nutrition for the rest of their life. It is very difficult for health care professionals to really understand what patients, clients and carers experience when they are prescribed long-term nutritional support via tube. Patients on Intravenous and Nasogastric Nutrition Therapy (PINNT) is a registered charity which aims to support both adults and children who require nutrition therapy (Activity 11.4).

Evaluation

The final stage of the process of nutritional care is evaluation of the care given. Student nurses should report 'to other members of the team when' the 'agreed plan is not achieved' (NMC 2007, p. 22). Nurses are expected to monitor and record progress against the plan of care to enable evaluation of the care given (NMC 2007, p. 22). Evaluation involves observation of the patient's/client's clinical condition and undertaking further screening or assessment of their nutritional status. Nurses should discuss progress and changes in the patient's/client's condition with the MDT (NMC 2007). It is important that the nurse 'reports malnutrition/worsening nutritional status as an adverse event and initiates appropriate action' (NMC 2007, p. 22). Finally, the nurse should challenge others who do not follow procedures (NMC 2007).

Ethical and Legal Issues

The provision of nutritional care can sometimes present complex ethical issues. Nurses must have an understanding of the ethical and legal issues relating to the provision and withdrawal of nutritional support. A review of these issues has been published recently by Körner *et al.* (2006). You may also want to read more about ethical and legal issues in Chapter 9 of this book.

Conclusion

This chapter has briefly reviewed the principles of nutritional science that are relevant to the provision of nutritional care by nurses and considered nutritional screening and assessment, care planning, nutritional interventions and evaluation of care planned. Nurses must ensure that patients/clients have their nutritional needs identified and a plan of care developed with other members of the MDT as required. The nurse is responsible for ensuring that the plan of nursing care is followed and evaluated, and that interventions undertaken follow local guidelines.

References

Age Concern (2006) *Hungry to be Heard*. Age Concern, London.

AHA (2006) *High Protein Diets*. American Heart Association, Dallas, online 2 April 2008, http://www.americanheart.org/presenter.jhtml?identifier=11234.\

BAPEN (British Association for Parenteral and Enteral Nutrition) (1996) *Standards and Guidelines for Nutritional Support of Patients in Hospitals*. British Association for Parenteral and Enteral Nutrition, Maidenhead.

BAPEN (British Association for Parenteral and Enteral Nutrition) (1999) *Current Perspectives on Enteral Nutrition in Adults*. British Association for Parenteral and Enteral Nutrition, Maidenhead.

BAPEN (British Association for Parenteral and Enteral Nutrition) (2006) *Malnutrition Universal Screening Tool: MUST*. BAPEN, Redditch (online), available at http://www.bapen.org.uk/pdfs/must/must_full.pdf

British Dietetics Association (2003) Effective Practice Bulletin, Issue 32. Challenging the use of Body Mass Index (BMI) to assess under-nutrition in older people. *Dietetics Today* 38(3): 15–19.

Brownie S. (2006) Why are elderly individuals at risk of nutritional deficient? *International Journal of Nursing Practice* 12: 110–118.

Davidson A., Scholefield H. (2005) Protecting mealtimes. *Nursing Management* 12(5): 32–36.

Dougherty L., Lister S. (2008) *The Royal Marsden Hospital Manual of Clinical Nursing Procedures*. Blackwell, Oxford.

Food Standards Agency (FSA) (2003) *Safe Upper Levels for Vitamins and Minerals*. Food Standards Agency Publications, London.

Food Standards Agency (FSA) (2007) *Eatwell Plate*, available on line at http://www.foodstandards.gov.uk/healthiereating/eatwellplate/

Food Standards Agency (FSA) (2008) *Healthy Diet*, available at http://www.eatwell.gov.uk/healthydiet/eighttipssection/; http://www.eatwell.gov.uk/agesandstages/

Green S.M., Watson R. (2005) Nutritional screening and assessment tools for use by nurses: literature review. *Journal of Advanced Nursing* 50(1): 69–83.

Körner U., Bondolfi A., Bühler E., MacFie J., Meguid M.M., Messing B., Oehmichen F., Valentini L., Allison S.P. (2006) Ethical and legal aspects of enteral nutrition. *Clinical Nutrition* 35: 196–202.

Lean M.E.J. (2000) Pathophysiology of obesity. *Proceedings of the Nutrition Society* 59: 331–336.

McLaren S., Green S. (1998) Nutritional screening and assessment. *Professional Nurse* (Study Supplement) 13(6): S9–S14.

NICE/National Collaborating Centre for Acute Care (2006) *Nutrition Support in Adults: Oral Nutrition Support, Enteral Tube Feeding and Parenteral Nutrition*. National Collaborating Centre for Acute Care, London, available at http://www.nice.org.uk/page.aspx?o=cg032

National Patient Safety Agency (2005) *How to Confirm the Correct Position of Nasogastric Feeding Tubes in Infants, Children and Adults.* NPSA, London, available at http://www.npsa. nhs.uk/patientsafety/alerts-and-directives/alerts/nasogastric-feeding-tubes/

Nursing and Midwifery Council (NMC) (2007) *Essential Skills Clusters.* NMC Circular 07 (2007) Annexe 2, NMC, London.

Nursing and Midwifery Council (NMC) (2008) *The Code: Standards of Conduct, Performance and Ethics for Nurses and Midwives.* NMC, London.

CHAPTER 12

Principles of Fluid Management

Michelle Denise Cowen

Introduction

This chapter provides you with the underpinning knowledge to adequately meet a patient's/client's fluid requirements. To help your understanding you will also need to read the relevant chapter(s) in your preferred physiology textbook. It may be helpful to keep this alongside you as you read this chapter.

The specific learning outcomes addressed in this chapter link with the Nursing and Midwifery Council's (NMC 2007) Essential Skills Clusters, and are identified below.

Learning outcomes

By the end of this chapter you will be able to do the following:

- Discuss why an adequate fluid intake is essential for survival.
- Identify what our fluid requirements are and how these change as a result of ill health or other factors.
- Identify factors which may affect an individual's ability to meet his or her fluid requirements.
- Discuss the importance of accurately measuring and recording fluid intake and output.
- Describe how to recognise signs of inadequate or excessive fluid intake.
- Discuss how an adequate fluid intake may be maintained when the individual is unable to do so by natural means.

Water – A Basic Human Need

To stay healthy, and indeed survive, our bodies are dependent on an adequate supply of food, oxygen and water. In fact, water is the most abundant chemical substance in our bodies and accounts for up to 60% of our body weight.

The majority of this water, a staggering 28 litres (67%) is contained within our cells and is known as intracellular fluid (ICF), the remainder is extracellular (ECF) and is split between interstitial fluid (24% or 10.5 litres) and intravascular fluid (8% or 3.5 litres). The final 1% is described as transcellular fluid and includes specialised body fluids such as cerebrospinal fluid (CSF), aqueous and vitreous humour within the eye, and lubricating fluids within joints and body organs.

Without water the body would be unable to fulfil its many functions and ultimately the person would die. Water is involved in processes such as the transportation of nutrients, electrolytes and blood gasses to the cells and contributes towards efficient removal of waste products, including metabolic wastes. In addition, it acts as a cushion, protecting the body organs from shock, provides a form of insulation and lubricates our cells and organs. Finally, it is essential to many chemical processes within the body, including the hydrolysis of food and the transfer of heat and electrical currents.

Further details on all of these functions are contained within any good physiology book and in order to enhance your understanding you should review these before reading any further.

The exact quantity of fluid within our body varies across the age continuum and between the sexes. As the bulk of the fluid within our body is contained within the muscles, men have a higher percentage with approximately 60% of their body weight being water. Women, due to a higher body fat content, and reduced muscle bulk have approximately 50% of their body weight comprising of water.

Age also plays an important part. *Newborn infants* may have as much as 70–80% of their body weight as water with 40% as extracellular fluid, which is a significantly higher ratio than in an adult. This coupled with a relatively larger quantity of fluid being ingested and secreted, results in the infant exchanging approximately half of their extracellular fluid volume each day, compared to approximately one-sixth in an adult (Metheny 2000). This leaves infants particularly vulnerable to fluid deficits as proportionately they have a much smaller reserve.

Older adults may also be at risk of fluid depletion. As muscle mass decreases with age, the total body fluid volume decreases to between 40% and 45% of body weight. This with changes in renal function and a reduction in the sensation of thirst (both of which will be discussed later in this chapter) place older adults at risk of fluid depletion and thus particularly susceptible to dehydration.

Daily fluid requirements

How much water do we need to maintain health? How does the body control input and output? Each day our body gains and loses fluids by various means with intake and output being roughly equal. Table 12.1 shows approximate volumes taken in and lost from different routes. The values indicated relate to a healthy adult and may vary significantly as a result of ill health.

Abnormal fluid loss

Diarrhoea may significantly increase the amount of fluid lost in the faeces, whilst pyrexia will bring about a dramatic increase in insensible loss. Additional losses from abnormal outputs such as wounds or vomit may also lead to a significant

Table 12.1   Daily water balance. *Source*: Marieb and Hoehn (2007).

Intake	Output
Drinks 1500 ml	Urine 1500 ml
Food 750 ml	Insensible loss (skin/lungs) 700 ml
Metabolism 250 ml	Sweat 200 ml
	Faeces 100 ml
Total taken in 2500 ml	Total output 2500 ml

fluid deficit if not replaced. In certain disease states the amount taken in may need to be restricted, for example for those patients with renal or cardiac failure. This may present particular difficulties for the persons concerned and it is therefore essential that they really enjoy what drinks they are allowed.

Maintaining Homeostasis

Key physiological processes help to control our fluid intake and output and thereby maintain homeostasis. A sign of early dehydration is thirst. The sensation of thirst is triggered by specialised cells, situated in the hypothalamus, known as osmoreceptors which are extremely sensitive to changes in the plasma osmolarity and respond accordingly. Hence thirst is a natural response to fluid depletion, and assuming that we have access to adequate fluids, by drinking to quench our thirst we can replace fluid loss to maintain homeostasis. However, if we are unable to drink adequate amounts to restore our body fluid, the body has another key process designed to keep us healthy. It conserves fluid within the body by secreting antidiuretic hormone (ADH) and aldosterone which reduces the amount of urine produced. It may be useful to explore these processes in your chosen physiology textbook as a good understanding is essential to detect abnormalities quickly.

Barriers to good hydration

Although the need for an adequate fluid intake is clear, there is now a wealth of evidence to suggest that many of our patients/clients are not receiving sufficient intake to maintain health (National Patient Safety Agency 2002). Helping patients maintain adequate fluid intake is therefore a fundamental role of the nurse.

One of the main reasons for an inadequate fluid intake is the lack of access to a drink when desired. For fit healthy adults this is unlikely to be a problem; however, if the individual has reduced mobility and/or dexterity it may be a significant obstacle. This may be as a result of age, illness or other mobility difficulties. Older adults living alone may be unable to prepare a drink for themselves, or carry it to where they wish to sit. The same could apply to individuals convalescing after surgery or debilitated by ill health. It is therefore essential that nurses take steps to ensure that drinks are always available and accessible. This includes pouring drinks for those unable to do so and placing them within reach and in a suitable drinking vessel. Safety is paramount and the use of specialised cups and/or straws may mean that an individual is able to maintain independence without risk of injury.

Poor fluid intake may also be due to a reduced desire to drink. Lukewarm water which has sat in a jug all day is unlikely to encourage anyone to drink. It is a fundamental part of the role of the nurse to find out what types of drink the individual likes and if possible to ensure that these are available, unless contraindicated for any medical reason. Cold, fresh water is much more palatable than that at room temperature and the addition of ice, if available, may make it even more so. Insulated jugs, often with a pushbutton dispenser, allow easy access to hot or cold drinks for several hours (Activity 12.1).

Activity 12.1

Look around the clinical environment when you are next in practice. What percentage of the patients/clients have a drink within reach? Ask them if they were given a choice and if the drink available is what they really want. Are they likely to drink it?

Physiological factors may also contribute to a reduced intake. In the older adult the sensation of thirst is diminished, reducing the desire to drink. Furthermore, a reduction in sodium levels and reduced kidney function will affect the sensitive fluid and electrolyte balance and reduce the body's ability to conserve fluids when necessary. Swallowing difficulties associated with a range of health problems may further contribute to worsening dehydration.

Recording and reporting fluid status

A fundamental role of the nurse is to ensure that all patients/clients receive adequate fluids to meet their daily needs. It is therefore essential that patients'/clients' fluid status is recorded accurately and information passed on to other members of staff where appropriate.

For the majority of patients/clients there are no significant variations on 'normal' daily requirements; however, for the reasons discussed earlier, some individuals may be unable to meet these needs unaided. Alongside the need for good basic nursing care is a requirement to closely monitor and record fluid intake through the use of a food and fluid records (see Chapter 11). This will allow the multidisciplinary team (MTD) involved in the individual's care, to review hydration by providing a record of the exact amount and type of fluid consumed that day.

Complex care

For other patients/clients, with more complex health care needs, a more detailed record, a *fluid balance chart* (FBC) will be required. FBCs record the volume and type of fluid taken in each day recording oral, entral, intravenous and subcutaneous fluids where appropriate. Fluid output is also carefully measured and recorded, with columns to record urinary output, vomit, nasogastric drainage/aspirate, faecal output/diarrhoea and drainage from wounds. This will allow the

> ### Activity 12.2
>
> Try discussing this with your mentor and discover the method used to measure and document quantities within your Trust area.

nurse to calculate the total in each column at the end of each 24-hour period and the overall balance (Activity 12.2).

Both food/fluid records and the more detailed FBCs are legal documents and should be carefully and meticulously completed. They not only act as a vital record of what the patients/clients have received but are key communication tools within the MTD. Despite this, there is a wealth of evidence to demonstrate that they are often not completed accurately and that this may, in some cases, contribute to increased patient morbidity and even mortality (Reid *et al.* 2004).

Assessing Fluid Status

A comprehensive assessment will include a 'look', 'listen' and 'feel' approach where the nurse considers the patient's/client's history, a visual assessment of observable clinical signs and measurement of objective clinical data. Together these form a 'jigsaw type picture' where the nurse should constantly be looking to see if each piece of information reinforces what is already known or differs, and may point in a different direction. It is essential that nothing is disregarded, however out of keeping it is with the overall picture, but is set aside and reconsidered periodically as the situation changes. It is important to remember that any type of assessment is an ongoing process, through which the nurse builds up a picture and constantly reviews this in the light of new information.

Accurate *history taking* is vital and the primary source of information are the patients/clients themselves, or if they are unable to communicate, their carer. Listening to what patients and carers say is crucial not only to assess their needs but to inform planning of truly individualised care. When taking a history it is important to consider the questions highlighted in Box 12.1.

> ### BOX 12.1
> ### Key questions in history taking
>
> - What would be considered to be a desirable fluid intake and output based on the assessment and the patient's/client's size, gender and age?
> - Has the person been able to meet this need? Can they drink unaided? Are they sufficiently mobile to get a drink at regular intervals and so on?
> - Do they have any health problems that are contributing to the amount of fluid loss and thereby increasing fluid requirements, for example pyrexia, diarrhoea, haemorrhage?
> - Are they on any medication that will affect their fluid balance, for example diuretics?
> - Have any fluid or dietary restrictions been prescribed that will impact on their fluid balance, for example, a low sodium diet or fluid restriction?
> - Are they generally in a positive, negative or neutral balance? Consider their cumulative FBC over the past few days.

In addition to obtaining a detailed history it is important that the nurse considers observable clinical signs to continue to build up the 'picture'. In order to do this an understanding of what signs to look for and how they might have changed in response to physiological processes is essential. Furthermore, knowing what other factors might cause these changes, and thereby distort the information demonstrates sound application of theoretical knowledge to practice. Table 12.2

Table 12.2 Observable parameters and their meaning.

Clinical signs/symptoms	Clinical significance	Cautions in interpretation
Mucous membranes will appear dry and the person will complain of thirst	Decreased saliva production will result in a dry mouth and sensation of thirst	Mouth breathing, oxygen administration, anticholinergic drugs
	Osmoreceptors detecting hypovolaemia will also trigger a feeling of thirst. This acts as a useful backup, as good mouth care often disguises the decreased saliva production	
Tongue furrows	A normal tongue has one long longitudinal furrow, but in dehydration additional furrows will be present and the tongue will appear smaller due to fluid loss (Lapides *et al.* 1965)	
Sunken eyes	As a result of decreased intra-ocular pressure	
Increased jugular venous pressure (JVP)	Distended veins indicate fluid overload	
With the person at 45° venous distension should not exceed 2cm above the sternal angle	Flat veins indicate decreased plasma volume	Assessing the right internal jugular vein gives a more reliable reading than on the left as it is the most anatomically direct route to the right atrium
Reduced capillary refill time	Capillary refill taking 2–3 seconds indicates a mild fluid deficit	Peripheral shutdown due to cold will slow capillary refill irrespective of fluid status
	Refill times in excess of 3 seconds signify severe fluid deficits	
Reduced skin turgor	Reduction in interstitial and intracellular fluid will reduce skin elasticity	In an older person it is difficult to detect changes in skin turgor due to the gradual loss of skin elasticity with age

(Continued)

Table 12.2   Continued.

Clinical signs/symptoms	Clinical significance	Cautions in interpretation
Cool peripheral temperature and pale skin colour	As a result of the renin/angiotensin cycle, hypovolaemia will result in peripheral vasoconstriction and therefore reduced temperature and colour	Individuals with poor circulation (e.g. peripheral vascular disease/Raynards disease) will normally have cool peripheries Certain antihypertensive drugs including vasodilators and ACE inhibitors will disguise the body's normal compensatory mechanism
Dark urine colour	Hypovolaemia will trigger release of anti-diuretic hormone, leading to more concentrated urine	Individuals with liver disease may have bilirubin present in their urine giving it a very dark colour Administration of diuretics will override the body's production of ADH
Peripheral oedema	Oedema occurs as a result of movement of fluid into interstitial spaces This can be as a result of fluid excess and/or reduced levels of plasma proteins A consequent decrease in intravascular fluid may lead to a drop in blood pressure	
Pulmonary oedema, observable through frothy sputum and/or shortness of breath	Pulmonary oedema will result in decreased gaseous exchange, with a reduction in oxygen saturations and arterial oxygen levels	

Based on a table originally published in Gobbi M.O., Cowen M.D., Ugboma D. (2006) Fluids and electrolytes. In: *Nursing Practice: Hospital and Home: The Adult*, 3rd edn. (eds Alexander M.F., Fawcett J.N., Runciman P.J.). Churchill Livingstone, Edinburgh, pp. 763–785.

identifies signs and symptoms of fluid depletion and overload that you need to look out for.

The final stage of collating information is the recording of objective clinical data. Ability to link these to the underpinning physiological processes is fundamental and you may find it helpful to have your favourite physiology textbook at hand. Table 12.3 outlines the most commonly performed clinical measurements made by the nurse, and again suggests the most likely cause, before drawing attention to alternative causes which might distort the picture (Activity 12.3).

Alternative measures may be used to assess fluid balance, which are considered by many to be more reliable and valid indicators. These include daily weight measurements, where the person is weighed at the same time each day using the same set of scales and wearing similar clothes/shoes. As lean body mass does not change

Table 12.3   Measurable parameters and their meaning.

Clinical measurements	Clinical significance	Cautions in interpretation
Pulse	If there is a reduction in circulating volume and therefore stroke volume, the heart rate will increase to compensate and maintain cardiac output	Cardiac drugs such as beta blockers will inhibit the body's compensatory mechanism and therefore block an increase in heart rate
	Initial assessment of rhythm, based on the regularity of the pulse, may be useful and indicate a need for an ECG recording	Pulse rate should be compared to the normal for the individual taking into account age and other influencing factors
Blood pressure	Measurement of blood pressure will give an idea of circulating volume	As a result of numerous compensatory mechanisms, blood pressure is maintained by the body for as long as possible. A 'normal' blood pressure in the presence of compensation must be acted upon immediately
	Pulse pressure (the difference between systolic and diastolic pressure) will give an indication of vasoconstriction i.e. compensation by the body	
Central venous pressure (CVP)	Will be reduced as a result of hypovolaemia and/or vasodilatation	
	An increase in CVP does not necessarily indicate fluid overload as CVP is influenced by numerous other factors including cardiac competence, systemic vascular resistance, intra-thoracic pressure and intra-abdominal pressure	
Urine volume	In health, the body produces 2 ml urine/kg of body weight/h up to the age of approximately 2 years. Thereafter it produces 1 ml urine/kg/h	A knowledge of the persons weight and calculation of desired urine output based upon that is essential
	Acceptable urine output in a critically ill patient is therefore equal to 0.5 ml urine/kg/h (or 1 ml/kg/h up to the age of 2)	Administration of diuretics will override normal physiological processes. Their use must be noted when assessing volume of urine produced
Specific gravity of urine	Demonstrates the body's ability to concentrate urine as an indicator of kidney function and/or response to ADH production	Administration of diuretics will override normal physiological processes. Their use must be noted when assessing urinary specific gravity

> **Activity 12.3**
>
> Select a patient/client that you have been involved in caring for and using the guidance questions on history taking and information in Tables 12.2 and 12.3, carry out an in-depth assessment of their fluid status.

very quickly any alterations are likely to be attributed to alterations in body fluid levels (Gobbi *et al.* 2006) Finally, bioelectrical impedance analysis (BIA) may be used where available (Metheny 2000). This involves passing an imperceptible electrical current through the person's body fluids by means of surface electrodes applied to his or her hand and foot. The extent to which the body conducts electricity can be used to estimate fluid volumes. A study by Mequid *et al.* (1992) found that BIA provided better correlation with FBCs than did daily weight measurements. Conclusions were that the speed and simplicity of this technique make it a valuable assessment tool. Despite this it is not commonly used in practice and further studies into its value may be beneficial to assess its potential to overcome the problems associated with assessing and recording fluid balance.

Fluid Replacement Therapy

So far the chapter has identified why fluids are essential to life and the potential causes of fluid deficits. Focus has been given to recognising the signs of dehydration or fluid overload. This underpinning knowledge allows the nurse to assess if the patient/client has the potential, with support and encouragement, to meet his or her fluid requirements, or if fluid replacement therapy is required. In most cases prescribing fluid replacement has been a doctor's role but with extended nurse practice and nurse prescribing, nurses are taking more responsibility for this. All nurses must be aware of the indications, requirements and associated risk of this commonly encountered therapy. Fluid replacement may be indicated where the patients/clients are unable to meet their fluid requirements orally, for whatever reason including cases of major fluid/electrolyte loss. The most commonly used route is intravenous (IV) administration, although subcutaneous (SC) administration (see subsection on Poor venous access) is gaining in popularity.

The IV route

The IV route is used to administer sterile fluid directly into a vein. In order to meet the intake normally obtained by drinking and eating, an adult would require approximately 2250 ml every 24 hours. However, additional fluid requirements to compensate for increased losses may dramatically increase this requirement and it is important to continue to assess for signs of dehydration/overload.

Different types of IV fluids are available and these are broadly categorised as crystalloids and colloids. Crystalloids are balanced salt solutions which diffuse quickly into the interstitial fluid and into the cells. Colloids are much more complex solutions with high molecular weights. The nature of the molecules contained within colloids makes them less able to diffuse out of the blood stream, providing

Section 4

Table 12.4 Commonly used IV fluids.

Intravenous fluid	Type	Features
Dextrose 5%	Crystalloid (isotonic)	• Commonly used for maintenance • Used to replace minor fluid loss • Provides some calorific value (small)
Normal saline	Crystalloid (isotonic)	• Commonly used for maintenance • Used to replace minor fluid loss • Used to correct hyponatraemia
Hartmans	Crystalloid (hypertonic)	• Used for maximum fluid and electrolyte replacement • Contraindicated in renal or hepatic disease
Blood – packed cells	Colloid (hypertonic)	• Used to replace red blood cells following major haemorrhage
Fresh frozen plasma	Colloid (hypertonic)	• Used to correct coagulation deficits
Gelofusine	Colloid (isotonic)	• Gelatine-based plasma expander • Short intravascular half-life • Carries significant risk of anaphylaxis from a toxic metabolite produced from gelatine synthesis
Hespan, HAES-steril, hydroxyethyl starch (HES)	Starch-based colloids	• Very high molecular weights • Extremely long half-life

---

Activity 12.4

During your next clinical practice placement look at what types of fluids patients are receiving and discuss with your mentor why that fluid was selected.

---

some degree of haemodynamic stability. The value of crystalloids above colloids and vice versa is still strongly debated, with various accounts and Cochrane reviews failing to agree on a definitive recommendation. However, for routine maintenance of fluid balance crystalloids remain the preferred group. Table 12.4 highlights the properties of the most commonly used IV fluids (Activity 12.4).

Care of a patient with an IV infusion

When caring for a patient/client with an IV infusion, certain procedures need to be observed. Observance of strict aseptic technique when changing the bag of fluid or dealing with the giving set or cannulae is essential. The potential for direct access of bacteria into the blood stream cannot be ignored. Research has shown that a bag of IV fluid should be changed every 24 hours, even when running very slowly and the giving set changed every 72 hours. Lines being used to administer parentral nutrition must be changed even more frequently – current recommendations are to change every 24 hours (Dougherty & Lister 2006). However, local policy may require more frequent changes, particularly if bolus injections of drugs are used in the giving set, and therefore local Trust policy must be adhered to.

Fluids must also be administered at the correct speed and the total volume infused recorded on the FBC. Fluids administered either too quickly or too slowly, may have profound effects on the patient's/client's well-being. Furthermore, failure to administer fluids in accordance with the prescribed rate constitutes a drug error as the prescription has not been adhered to and must be reported. For more information on drug errors read the section on Safety and Governance Structures in Chapter 14 of this book.

Fluids are routinely administered via an *infusion pump* to control the rate of delivery; however, it is essential that the nurse is able to calculate the number of drops per minute to be infused in case a pump is not available and for safety reasons. The standard formula is

$$\text{Flow rate (drops/min)} = \frac{\text{Volume of fluid to be infused (ml)}}{\text{Infusion time (min)} \times \text{drop factor}}$$

The drop factor is stated on the giving set wrapper, but for standard giving sets it is 20 drops per ml for crystalloids and 15 drops per ml for colloids. For micro-drop sets (where the fluid drops through a needle into a burette) the drop factor is 60 drops per ml (Activity 12.5).

Activity 12.5

Calculate the following infusion rates, first as a rate to set on an infusion pump and then in terms of drips per minute if a pump is not available.

1. 1000 ml saline over 8 hours through a standard giving set
2. 500 ml dextrose over 6 hours through a micro-drop set
3. 250 ml gelofusine through a standard giving set

Whether fluid is being administered intravenously or subcutaneously the insertion site needs to be checked regularly for signs of complications. These are summarised in Table 12.5.

Poor venous access

For older adults with poor venous access, confused patients and for some terminally ill patients, the preferred route of administration is subcutaneous (Mansfield & Monaghan Hall 1998). The sites of choice are the abdominal wall, anterior or lateral aspects of the chest wall, anterolateral aspects of the thigh and finally the scapula. Fluid is administered via a butterfly needle at a maximum rate of 2 litres in 24 hours. The administration site should be inspected regularly and changed on a 24-hour basis. An advantage of this route is that fluid can be administered overnight and the butterfly needle removed during the day to facilitate mobility and promote independence. Careful documentation of which site has been used each time will prevent the reuse of a site too quickly to maintain skin integrity and minimise risk of infection.

Section 4

Table 12.5   Complications of IV fluid administration.

Complication	Explanation/actions
Phlebitis	Localised redness and tenderness along the route of the vein, caused by the presence of the cannulae or from the substances infused. Cannulae needs to be resited
Infiltration	Infusion of fluid into the tissues resulting in localised swelling/discomfort. Cannulae needs to be resited
Extravasation	Infusion of irritant substances into the tissues, often resulting in severe tissue damage and necrosis. Stop infusion immediately and seek specialised advice
Infection	Localised infection around cannulae site. Cannuale needs to be resited. Antibiotic treatment may be required
Septicaemia	Serious systemic infection as a result of pathogenic bacteria being directly introduced into the blood stream. Urgent medical attention required
Fluid overload	Caused when fluid is administered too rapidly or in too great a quantity. Urgent medical assessment required
Fluid deficit	Caused when fluid is administered too slowly or in insufficient volume. Medical review required
Emboli	Caused when a blood clot is dislodged from the cannulae site and enters the systemic circulation

Conclusion

This chapter has highlighted the fundamental need for water in order for our bodies to stay healthy. It identifies the vast quantities of fluid contained within our cells, tissues and blood stream, making up approximately 50–60% of our total body weight. Basic daily requirements and homeostatic mechanisms used to control intake and output are explored to provide a sound foundation for developing essential nursing skills. Most importantly, this chapter seeks to raise awareness of barriers to maintaining adequate hydration and explore ways of overcoming these. Recognising signs of fluid depletion or overload are fundamental to helping to meet patients'/clients' needs. A significant proportion of the chapter was therefore devoted to helping you to develop your knowledge and skills in this aspect of assessment. Finally, ways of providing adequate hydration to those will aid your understanding unable to drink were explored along with the associated nursing care (Activity 12.6).

Section 4

Activity 12.6

Further reading and resources

Alderson P., Schierhout G., Roberts I., Bunn F. (2003) *Colloids Versus Crystalloids for Fluid Resuscitation in Critically Ill Patients* (*Cochrane review*). The Cochrane Library, Issue 4. Wiley, Chichester.

Lippincott, Williams and Wilkins (2008) *Fluids and Electrolytes Made Incredibly Easy,* 4th edn. Lippincott, Williams and Wilkins, Philadelphia.

Marieb E.N., Hoehn K. (2007) *Human Anatomy and Physiology*, 7th edn. Pearson, San Francisco.

References

Dougherty L., Lister S.E. (2006) *The Royal Marsden Hospital Manual of Clinical Nursing Procedures*. Blackwell, Oxford.

Gobbi M.O., Cowen M.D., Ugboma D. (2006) Fluids and electrolytes. In: *Nursing Practice: Hospital and Home: The Adult,* 3rd edn. (eds Alexander M.F., Fawcett J.N., Runciman P.J.). Churchill Livingstone, Edinburgh.

Lapides J., Bourne R., Maclean L. (1965) Clinical signs of dehydration and extracellular fluid loss. *Journal of American Medical Association* 191: 413.

Mansfield S., Monaghan Hall J. (1998) Subcutaneous administration and site maintenance. *Nursing Standard* 13(12): 56–62.

Marieb E.N., Hoehn K. (2007) *Human Anatomy and Physiology*, 7th edn. Pearson, San Francisco.

Metheny N.M. (2000) *Fluid and Electrolyte Balance. Nursing Considerations*, 4th edn. Lippincott, Philadelphia.

Mequid M., Lukaski H., Tripp M., Rosenburg J., Parker F. (1992) Rapid bedside method to assess changes in postoperative fluid status with bioelectrical impedance analysis. *Surgery* 112: 502.

National Patient Safety Agency (2002) *National Reporting Goes Live*. www.npsa.nhs.uk

Nursing and Midwifery Council (NMC) (2007) *Essential Skills Clusters*. NMC Circular 07(2007) Annexe 2, NMC, London.

Reid J., Robb E., Stone D., Bowen P, Baker R., Irving S., Waller M. (2004) Improving the monitoring and assessment of fluid balance. *Nursing Times* 100(20): 36–39.

Section 5

Medicines Management

CHAPTER 13

Principles of Pharmacology

Jane Caroline Portlock

Introduction

This chapter introduces you to medicines, how they work, how they are used therapeutically and how they are regulated. It is complementary to Chapter 14 and the two are designed to interact with each other.

The specific learning outcomes addressed in this chapter link with the Nursing and Midwifery Council's (NMC 2007) Essential Skills Clusters, and are identified below.

Learning outcomes

By the end of this chapter you will be able to do the following:

- Describe how medicines work in the human body (pharmacology).
- Describe how the human body affects medicines (pharmacokinetics).
- Identify how illness and the extremes of age can affect how the body handles medicines.
- Demonstrate where information about medicines can be found and how this information can be applied in practice.
- Describe the legal, ethical and professional aspects of the regulation of medicines.
- Illustrate the application of evidence-based practice for the drug treatment of diabetes within a Therapeutic Framework.

A Therapeutic Framework activity is presented as a tool for organising learning about the use of medicines for common conditions. The suggested activities will enable you to structure your learning and develop your own Therapeutic Framework for wherever you are in clinical practice.

What are Medicines?

Medicines are commonly used to treat patients' conditions. Increasingly potent and sophisticated treatment regimens mean that people can often be prescribed three or more medicines for a single medical condition. Even modern medicines are not without side effects, so care needs to be taken, when looking after patients, to consider whether the medicines they are taking are causing problems or are ineffective. Side effects and perceived risks can cause the patients to stop taking their medicines. Adverse effects which are missed by those caring for patients can cause harm. However, many medicines have a huge, positive impact on a disease, offering a cure or halting the progression of the condition. Therefore, it is important to be aware of the impact which medicines have, in terms of successful treatment and side effects. Medicines are licensed for use in the United Kingdom by the Medicines and Healthcare Products Regulatory Agency. Information on their therapeutic use, dose regimen, cautions and contraindications can be found in the *British National Formulary* (BNF 2008) which should be available to all health care professionals who are looking after patients.

More detailed product information is available from the Summary of Product Characteristics (SPCs) which can be found on-line at www.medicines.org.uk the website of the Medicines and Healthcare products Regulatory Agency (MHRA). SPCs include details of name and composition of product, pharmaceutical formulation, therapeutic indications, method of administration, contraindication, special warnings and precautions for use, interactions, effects on pregnancy and lactation, undesirable effects including effects on ability to drive and operate machinery, pharmacodynamic and pharmacokinetic properties, preclinical safety date, incompatibilities, special precautions for storage, disposal and other handling and shelf life.

How Medicines Affect Patients – Pharmacology and Pharmacokinetics

Medicines (often called drugs) are chemicals which change what is happening in the body. Medicines almost always work by acting on target proteins. The target protein can be one of three main types: receptor, enzyme and ion channel. The term receptor means a protein molecule which recognises and responds to chemicals within the body. A medicine can mimic the body's own chemicals and trigger a response or can antagonise the body's chemicals and therefore slow down or even stop a normal function. Examples of the three main types of drug action include the following:

- salbutamol which is a beta 2 agonist and acts on beta 2 adrenaline receptors mainly in the lungs causing bronchodilation;
- non-steroidal anti-inflammatory drugs inhibit the enzyme cyclo-oxygenase which decreases the production of prostaglandins from arachidonic acid and therefore decreases inflammation and

- amlodipine which is a calcium channel blocker and stops calcium moving from the outside to the inside of the cell membrane of vascular smooth muscle therefore preventing contraction of the blood vessel which needs calcium (Rang & Dale 2007).

Pharmacokinetics describes what the body does to the medicine. Most drugs are given orally and are absorbed from the gut into the bloodstream. Some drugs can also be given intravenously (via a vein), subcutaneously (under the skin), intramuscularly (into a muscle) or transdermally (across the skin from a transdermal patch which adheres to the skin) so that the drug goes directly into the blood stream from the site of administration. The drug will then be distributed (carried around the body) and will reach the site(s) of action. The blood stream transports the drug to the liver, where it can be metabolised (broken down) into inactive components and the kidneys where water-soluble drugs (and water-soluble metabolites) can be excreted. The characteristics of the drug's absorption, distribution, metabolism and excretion can often be predicted from knowing the patient's renal (kidney) and liver (hepatic) function, weight and age.

The type of drug needed, dose and frequency of administration can be modified if these characteristics are taken into consideration. Drugs that have a narrow therapeutic index (where the toxic dose is only slightly higher than the therapeutic dose) have to be monitored very carefully, examples include digoxin, warfarin and phenytoin.

The phrase drug 'half-life' describes the time taken for the concentration of the drug in the blood to fall by half. It is often used to describe the elimination characteristics of the drug. Drugs with long half-lives persist in the body for longer, which increases the chances of toxicity. Drugs with short half-lives are rapidly excreted and need to be taken more frequently to sustain an effect. Application of pharmacokinetics helps in treatment, but the patient should be treated as a whole, with consideration of the potential effects of other conditions and drugs which can interact with each other (Walker & Whittlesea 2007).

How Patients Affect Medicines: Extremes of Age, Impact of Hepatic and Renal Insufficiency and Other Major Problems such as Heart Disease and Diabetes

Babies and children need careful consideration when being treated with medicines as their bodies do not behave as if they are small adults. Children and babies differ from adults in their response to drugs; the risk of toxicity is increased by a reduced rate of clearance from the body and higher organ sensitivity. Children's doses are often expressed in terms of amount of drug (e.g. dose in milligrams) per kilogram of ideal body weight of the child, or by a specific dose for body surface area (in metre^2). Body surface area estimates are usually more accurate for calculating doses than body weight because many functions within the body relate better to surface area than weight. Body surface area can be estimated from weight by means of the table printed inside the back cover of the BNF. Weight and surface area may change significantly within a short period of time. Where the dose is not stated for children or in cases of uncertainty, advice should be sought from a medicines information centre (BNF). It is important that the child and the child's carer are able to tell the difference between side effects (adverse effects) and the effects of the medical condition, so that they can report any problems.

The use of medicines in the elderly should also be given special attention. The most important effect of age is reduction in renal function, which results in the slowing down of excretion of medicines and greater potential for kidney damage by drugs toxic to the kidney. The metabolism of some medicines by the liver is also reduced in the older person. The concentration of drugs in the tissue may also increase, due to dehydration and decreased kidney function.

The guidelines for medicines use in the older person include limiting the range of medicines prescribed and simplifying the regimen so that medicines only need to be taken once or twice a day, reducing the dose of the medicine whenever possible, regularly reviewing the medicines being given, explaining clearly with full written instructions which can be read and understood and telling the patients what to do when medicines run out and making sure that matching quantities are prescribed so that they all run out at the same time, which simplifies the repeat prescription.

Liver (hepatic) disease may alter the response to medicines in a number of ways, but liver disease has to be severe before important changes in drug metabolism occur. Liver function tests do not predict how well drugs will be metabolised, so it is often quite difficult to predict what the dose should be reduced to. Other problems related to liver disease include reduced production of blood-clotting factors by the liver, impaired brain function due to build up of toxins, fluid overload and increased damage to the liver by drugs.

From Pharmacology to Therapeutics: Commonly Prescribed Drugs, What You should Know and Where to Look

The most important source of information on medicines is the BNF (2008). Any health care professional should have a current edition and be familiar with its contents. It provides a wide range of information from general advice on medicines, special considerations in medicines use such as renal or hepatic disease, pregnancy, breastfeeding, extremes of age and palliative care. It also provides a starting place for looking up drug interactions to check whether they are clinically important as well as information on wound management products, emergency treatment of poisoning and so on. The inside front cover contains useful telephone numbers including the NHS Medicines Information Services which can provide information on any aspect of drug therapy and are located around the country.

The main contents cover the individual drugs grouped according to which part of the body and condition they are used to treat. Each drug section has an introductory paragraph which provides general prescribing advice, usually a mention of the evidence-based guidelines, together with a description of any special precautions or monitoring which is required. Every licensed drug in the United Kingdom is included in the BNF. Under each specific drug heading there is a description of the indications (conditions) for which the drug is licensed, cautions (where the drug can be used with careful monitoring and/or reduced dose due to specific problems or other conditions from which the patient could be suffering), contraindications (specific conditions which prevent the use of the drug because it might harm the patient), side effects (untoward effects which need to be monitored for), dose in each specific condition, names (both proprietary/trade name and approved name), formulation (e.g. tablets, suspension, injection) and frequency of dosing.

Newer drugs which require special monitoring and reporting of all serious side effects will have a black triangle (▼) on the right of the trade and approved name (see section on Regulation of Medicines Use: Legal, Ethical and Professional Aspects of Drugs Regulation in this chapter). Drugs which have the symbol of a rectangle with a diagonal line bottom left to top right and the lower half shaded black are considered by the Joint Formulary Committee to be less suitable for prescribing. The use of these drugs is only very occasionally justifiable. The BNF is designed for rapid reference and may not always cover all the information necessary for appropriate use of the drug. Further information can be found in product literature (e.g. patient information leaflets included with the product), the SPCs (see the section on What are Medicines) and specialist literature such as evidence-based guidelines as well as by contacting Medicines Information (MI) centres around the United Kingdom. The BNF is also available on-line via www.bnf.org.

When nursing a patient who is taking any medicines, you should be familiar with the usual dose and frequency of administration of the medicine, together with information on possible side effects as well as the consequences to the patient of not taking the medicine. Adverse effects from drugs can be very important and can often cause the patient to suffer from confusion, falls and sedation, all of which can be mistakenly attributed to other factors when their medicines are, in fact, at the root of the problem. Patients can suffer serious harm due to medicine-related problems and as a consequence may be hospitalised, so the effects of the medicines they are taking should never be underestimated. Twenty of the most commonly prescribed drugs (NHS/PPD 2008) can be found in Box 13.1. This list gives a good idea of the sort of medicines you will commonly encounter and need to be familiar within clinical practice (Activity 13.1).

BOX 13.1

List of commonly prescribed drugs

bendroflumethiazide	aspirin	atenolol
paracetamol	salbutamol	furosemide
atorvastatin	levothyroxine	metformin
simvastatin	amoxicillin	lansoprazole
lactulose	fluoxetine	diclofenac
gliclazide	co-dydramol	co-codamol
amlodipine	omeprazole	

Activity 13.1

Why not make a data log of the above medicines and find out as much as you can about them so that you become very familiar with them. Access this information by visiting the website www.medicines.org.uk and the BNF website www.bnf.org.

Regulation of Medicines Use: Legal, Ethical and Professional Aspects of Drugs Regulation

No medicine is ever 100% safe, because all medicines have side/adverse effects. Different people respond to medicines differently. Several factors can influence the chances of side effects, including the prescribed dose, condition being treated, the age and the sex of the patient and other treatments which the patient may be taking, including herbal and other purchased remedies. Medicines are thoroughly tested on thousands of people and must meet rigorous standards before they are licensed. However, some side effects only come to light after use for a couple of years in thousands of patients. Therefore, medicines also need to be carefully monitored even after they have been granted a licence, in case anything adverse occurs. The MHRA is a government body which was set up in 2003 to continue the work of the Medicines Control Agency (MCA) which existed before then. The functions of the MHRA include regulation of medicines and the investigation of harmful incidents involving medicines which have already received a licence. The principal aim of the Agency is to safeguard the public by making sure that medicines work properly and are acceptably safe. If a concern does come to light the MHRA responds quickly to make a decision about the future of the drug or issues special advice to prevent the problem recurring.

A licence, also referred to as a marketing authorisation, is required before any medicine can be used to treat people in the United Kingdom. To begin the process of applying for a licence the pharmaceutical companies must apply to the MHRA for permission to test drugs through clinical trials. All the results from these trials are sent to the MHRA for detailed assessment. Once the MHRA is satisfied that the medicine works as it should, and that it is acceptably safe, it is given a product licence.

New medicines are put on probation for up to two years and labelled with a black triangle (▼) to ensure that prescribers and other people looking after the patient are aware of the need to monitor them carefully. The black triangle accompanies new medicines in product information, prescribing manuals and advertising material. It prompts health care professionals to report any potential side effects to the MHRA. This information helps to build up a broader picture of how the medicine works in the general population and enables the MHRA to act promptly if a previously unrecognised and serious side effect comes to light. The black triangle is not removed until the MHRA is satisfied that the medicine works safely in a large number of people.

There are a number of schemes to monitor patient safety, two of which are run by the MHRA. The first is the General Practice Research Database (GPRD) which contains thousands of anonymised patient records and is used to look for links between new symptoms which the patient reports, or are identified by the general practitioner (GP) and the medicines which the patient is taking. The database has already been used to see whether there were serious side effects associated with common treatments such as the oral contraceptive pill, hormone replacement therapy and antidepressants. The second scheme is the Yellow Card Scheme – a reporting system for possible side effects related to medicines. This scheme is available for patients, carers and all health care professionals to report suspicions that a medicine has caused a problem. The person reporting does not have to be convinced that there is a connection between the medicine and the adverse effect, nor does the adverse effect need to be previously unknown. The MHRA can sift through all of the data from these sources and make decisions about drug safety based on the large amount of data they receive. The Yellow Card Scheme receives over 20 000 reports of possible adverse effects every year, and it is hoped that by opening up the scheme to enable patients and carers the number of reports will increase still further to provide more information to enhance the safety of medicines. Only one medicine in every 25 000 is ever withdrawn as a result of a problem being identified. This demonstrates that the initial licensing procedure is thorough (Medicines and Healthcare Products Regulatory Agency n.d.).

Developing a Therapeutic Framework for Medicines Use: Introduction to Activity 13.2

The 'Therapeutic Framework' has been developed over nearly a decade to help students organise their knowledge of medicines and underpin the development of their skills. It is a useful way of organising all the information needed when looking after a patient with a particular condition and ensuring that the care is based on evidence and safe practice. There are ten steps to undertake in developing a 'Therapeutic Framework' (Box 13.2). Steps 1–5 consider the medicines-related issues and the patient. Steps 6–10 relate to practical aspects of medicines management and clinical governance (measures which can be taken to decrease risks to the patient from treatment).

BOX 13.2

The Therapeutic Framework

1. Pathophysiology of the disease (what has gone wrong in the body) and therapeutic use in a specific clinical condition (mode of action of drugs used to treat the disease).
2. Pharmacoepidemiology – pattern of disease and pattern of drug use – how common is the condition, which medicines are you likely to see used to treat the condition in your practice area?
3. Pharmacoeconomics – how much does it cost to treat the condition and what are the measures of benefit/effectiveness which can be measured?
4. Patient and clinical monitoring.
5. Evidence-based guidelines.
6. Medicines management issues.
7. Developing your medicines management role.
8. Clinical governance issues.
9. Where does medicines management for this group of patients fit into the NHS?
10. The team approach – how is the patient looked after, by whom and how does it all join up to enhance care?

Do not be put off by this list, each step is explained in detail below. Some steps will require information from textbooks and various websites, others will require discussion with patients and their carers and other members of the health care team (e.g. GPs, pharmacists, senior nurses, physiotherapists, occupational therapists, social workers). Your mentor will also be able to help you in all these areas. When writing a Therapeutic Framework, you can start anywhere, though it is often easier to work through it in numerical order.

Case study 13.1 provides an example of a completed Therapeutic Framework for non-insulin-dependent diabetes. You may want to read this through first before embarking on developing your own Therapeutic Framework in Activity 13.2.

Case study 13.1

Therapeutic Framework for a common condition – non-insulin-dependent diabetes (type two diabetes)

1. Pathophysiology of diabetes and mode of action of drugs

Insulin is a hormone secreted by the pancreas which increases energy stores during times of adequate nutrition and works together with other hormones (adrenaline, corticosteroids, glucagon and growth hormone) to mobilise glucose when energy use increases. Insulin has a wide range of effects on metabolism of carbohydrates, lipids and proteins. It enhances cellular uptake of glucose from the blood in many tissues particularly skeletal muscle and adipose tissue and as result reduces blood glucose levels. Non-insulin-dependent diabetes occurs when there is a relative deficiency of insulin or a resistance to insulin within the body. Treatment aims to correct the symptoms (tiredness, blurred vision, increased urine production, thirst) and achieve tight control over blood sugar levels. This will in turn prevent macrovascular and microvascular complications such as retinopathy, nephropathy and neuropathy. Diet is the first-line therapy to reduce the total body fat. Medicines are then included if diet alone is ineffective. The aim is to control blood glucose so that it is 4–10 mmol/litre. Sulphonylureas (e.g. gliclazide) work by augmenting insulin secretion but are only effective when residual pancreatic beta-cell function (which leads to insulin production) is present. Biguanides (e.g. metformin) inhibits hepatic gluconeogenesis (glucose production) and increases peripheral use of glucose. Acarbose inhibits alpha-glucosides enzyme in the intestines preventing the absorption of starch and sucrose. Repaglinide promotes the secretion of insulin by closing ATP-sensitive potassium channel in the beta-cell membrane. Glitazones (e.g. rosiglitazone) directly enhance insulin sensitivity which reduces insulin resistance. Insulin reduces blood glucose levels.

2. Pharmacoepidemiology – pattern of disease and pattern of drug use – how common is the condition, which medicines are you likely to see used to treat the condition in your practice area?

The estimated prevalence of diabetes in the United Kingdom is 3.5%, based on data from the GMS contract quality and outcomes framework. The incidence of diabetes has been estimated at 1.7 new diagnoses per 1000 persons per year (around 85 000 cases per year in England and 5000 cases per year in Wales). By the year 2010, the number of people with diabetes in the United Kingdom is predicted to reach 3 million. The prevalence of diabetes increases sharply with age. In the United Kingdom, 1 in 20 people over 65 years of age has diabetes, compared with 1 in 5 people over 85 years of age. Of people with diabetes, 90% have type two diabetes.

3. Pharmacoeconomics: how much does it cost to treat the condition and what are the measures of benefit/effectiveness which can be measured?

It is more cost effective to achieve better blood glucose levels by use of numerous medicines (treatment combinations) which will reduce the need for intensive medical care later on.

4. Patient and clinical monitoring

The following should be routinely monitored: cholesterol and triglyceride levels to check for hyperlipidaemia; blood glucose levels; HbA1c to monitor long-term control of blood glucose levels; urea and electrolytes plus serum creatinine to monitor renal function; liver function tests; thyroid function tests.

5. Evidence-based guidelines

The National Institute for Health and Clinical Excellence (NICE) guidelines 2002 state that the target HbA1c levels should be between 6.5% and 7.5%. Metformin is used as the first-line glucose lowering therapy for patients who are obese provided that they do not have renal failure. Sulphonylureas and repaglanide are used as first-line options when metformin is not tolerated or the patient is not obese. Metformin and sulphonylureas are used in combination with metformin in obese people when glucose control becomes unsatisfactory. Glitazones are used in combination with metformin or sulphonylureas (but not both) if the metformin/sulphonylurea combination is not tolerated. Insulin treatment is offered to patients who have inadequate blood glucose control on optimised oral medicine combinations.

6. Medicines management issues

Gastrointestinal intolerance is common when starting treatment with metformin, to minimise this effect, the dose should be increased slowly over several weeks. Metformin is contraindicated in people with renal impairment or cardiac failure. These people are at increased risk of lactic acidosis. Lactic acidosis is a rare, potentially fatal adverse effect of metformin therapy. Symptoms are non-specific to start with, such as malaise, respiratory distress and bradycardia. Hypoglycaemia is a recognised adverse effect of sulphonylureas. It is most likely to affect older people, especially those with worsening renal function. Major hypoglycaemia occurs in 1–2% of people receiving sulphonylureas. This group of drugs is mainly metabolised by the liver and then cleared by the kidneys. Impairment of hepatic and renal function increases the risk of hypoglycaemia. Weight gain (2–5 kg) is common with this group of drugs. It is recommended that people should have liver function tests before starting treatment with glitazones, then every two months for the first year and regularly after that. Treatment should stop when liver enzyme levels rise to above three times the normal upper limit. Glitazones are contraindicated in people with cardiac failure, because they can cause fluid retention. Patients should be monitored for signs and symptoms of heart failure. Use of non-steroidal anti-inflammatory drugs with this group of drugs can increase the risk of fluid retention. Glitazones are contraindicated in combination with insulin as an increased risk of heart failure has been observed. Glitazones are associated with significant weight gain, probably due to fluid retention. After starting treatment there may be a delay of 6–10 weeks before the full effect of glitazones is seen.

7. Developing your medicines management role

Compliance support is a big part of medicines management in diabetes. Lifestyle and dietary advice is important, but so is looking at the patient's motivation, readiness to make adjustments and helping him or her to adopt healthier lifestyles. Support for medicines taking is also vital, as is education and encouragement for blood glucose monitoring.

8. Clinical governance issues

Treatment should be regularly audited to check that guidelines are being followed. It is important to be familiar with the most recent evidence-based guidelines such as those provided by www.cks.library.nhs.uk. Critical incidents, errors and near misses should be reported to the National Patient Safety Agency www.npsa.nhs.uk. Adverse drug reactions should be reported to the MHRA via the yellow card scheme available at www.mhra.gov.uk. Local guidelines should be regularly reviewed (check for a review date before using any guideline) and be based on nationally available evidence.

9. Where does medicines management for this group of patients fit into the NHS?

Developments in the support of self-care, patient partnerships and self-management will all contribute to the enhancement of care for this group of patients. There is a National Service Framework for the care of patients with diabetes (DH 2001) which describes the strategy for the development of care and education for this group of patients.

10. The team approach – how is the patient looked after, by whom and how does it all join up to enhance care?

Diabetes care is almost always multidisciplinary, with protocols and guidelines for treatment and support. Different members of the team are aware of the scope of their and other members' roles and responsibilities. Medicines management responsibilities are shared between the team, with the patient getting clear, consistent information and support from everyone.

Activity 13.2

Complete your own Therapeutic Framework

Identify a common condition in the practice area in which you are working. Now complete the 10-step activities below to complete your own Therapeutic Framework. Keep the example Therapeutic Case study 13.1 close to hand, as this provides you with an excellent example of a completed framework for non-insulin diabetes.

Step 1: Activity 13.2.1

Pathophysiology of the disease (what has gone wrong in the body) and therapeutic use in a specific clinical condition (mode of action of drugs used to treat the disease)

Make short notes on the condition including information on aetiology (cause), pathophysiology (the problem within the body), and the pharmacology (mode of action of the drugs within the body) and pharmacokinetics (the way the body affects the absorption, distribution, metabolism and excretion) of the main drugs used to treat the condition. This will help you to familiarise yourself with the condition and ensure that you are clear about how the drugs actually work, before looking at more patient-related features and evidence-based aspects of therapeutics in the next sections. Consult your School of Nursing recommended textbooks for information on pathophysiology and pharmacology. It is worth looking at a number of publications before selecting the one most suited to your needs.

Step 2: Activity 13.2.2

Pharmacoepidemiology – pattern of disease and pattern of drug use: How common is the condition, which medicines are you likely to see used to treat the condition in your practice area?

Describe the prevalence of the disease: How common is it?

Note the main drug groups which are prescribed and the main medicines within each group. Identify patterns of prescribing and drug combinations that are commonly used, so that you are aware of local practice with medicines use for this condition. Compare what you actually see happening in practice with good evidence-based practice from published evidence and guidelines. Search for this information online via the NHS library www.library. nhs.uk and the Clinical Knowledge Summaries Service www.cks.library.nhs.uk.

Step 3: Activity 13.2.3

Pharmacoeconomics: How much does it cost to treat the condition and what are the measures of benefit/effectiveness?

Look up the cost of treatment in terms of cost per course and cost per month in your BNF. Describe the expected outcomes of treatment in terms of effectiveness of the medicine and the benefit to the patient. Sometimes cost/benefit information is available in published studies, which puts a monetary value on the outcomes of treatment. Non-drug costs (e.g. monitoring costs) also need to be identified. It is useful to know these figures, because prescribing decisions (e.g. such as whether or not to include a drug in a local formulary) consider this type of information. Access the following website to identify information on cost-effectiveness: www.nice.org.uk. Also check out www.npc.co.uk; the website of the National Prescribing Centre publishes the MeReC bulletins to summarise and explain the cost/effectiveness of new medicines.

Step 4: Activity 13.2.4

Patient and clinical monitoring: Identify how the patient is monitored and which tests are ordered

Make a note of the terminology and abbreviations associated with this therapeutic area. Convert the terms used to easy-to-understand words and phrases to enable you to explain all aspects of the treatment to the patient. The parameters which need to be measured should be described in this section. These fall into two categories – patient monitoring and clinical monitoring.

Patient monitoring – List the signs and symptoms of the condition, how it is diagnosed; are any diagnostic aids used and assessed throughout the treatment?

What would you ask the patient about their signs and symptoms while monitoring treatment?

What signs and symptoms would you need to monitor? Look out for both therapeutic benefits and any side/adverse effects of treatment).

Identify how you would determine successful outcome of treatment, no therapeutic benefit or deterioration of the condition.

Clinical monitoring refers to the measurement of blood and urine for specific components, such as potassium, sodium, creatinine, a full blood count and actual levels of drug, all of which can provide an indication of the effect of the drug on the body. Monitoring of renal and hepatic function is often necessary as well as other measures such as blood pressure, pulse, respiratory function, ECG (electrocardiogram) and so on. These parameters will be specific to the condition and treatment, so it is important to know what should be monitored and when. Information on patient and clinical monitoring is often summarised in the BNF, but further information should also be sought, by checking with the local, clinical guidelines, expert opinion and with the Summary of Product Characteristics (www.medicines.org.uk).

Access these listed resources to enable you to list all the patient and clinical monitoring required. Also check this out with your mentor.

Step 5: Activity 13.2.5

Evidence-based guidelines

Identify the relevant guidelines for this particular condition. Access the National Health and Clinical Excellence website for published guidelines – www.nice.org.uk as well as the Scottish Intercollegiate Guidelines Network www.sign.ac.uk and the evidence-based

guidelines published by the NHS Clinical Knowledge Summaries Service www.cks.library.
nhs.uk. Ask your mentor if any local guidelines are available. These are usually adapted from
national guidelines. Check out that any local guidance is based on current best evidence.

Step 6: Activity 13.2.6

Medicines management issues

List any issues which may affect how the patient takes the medicine. Are there any allergies,
adverse drug reactions, interactions? What range of formulations is available? (e.g. tablets,
suspension). Consider how compliance may be encouraged.

Identify self-management tools and the health promotion strategies indicated (Chapter 14
may help you here).

Step 7: Activity 13.2.7

Developing your medicines management role

Consider the nurses' role in caring for this group of patients, taking into account best practice. Discuss this with your mentor and consider how the nurse may extend practice, for
example, by prescribing for this group of patients.

Step 8: Activity 13.2.8

*Clinical governance issues: Consider risk reduction, how the patient's treatment is audited
and Continuing Professional Development (CPD)*

There are a number of clinical governance issues, but the key ones for the Therapeutic
Framework are audit, continuing professional development and risk reduction.

List how the patient's treatment is measured and audited.

What steps should be taken in the event of adverse events or error?

What further Continuing Professional Development (CPD) would be useful for the health
care practitioner in order to enhance the care of the patient?

There are several useful websites for this information including www.nelm.nhs.uk (the
National Electronic Library for medicine), www.npc.co.uk (the National Prescribing Centre)
and www.npsa.nhs.uk (the National Patient Safety Agency) see also the relevant sections in
Chapter 14.

Step 9: Activity 13.2.9

Where does medicines management for this group of patients fit into the NHS?

Identify the key NHS documents which relate to the particular condition.

Identify if there is a relevant National Service Framework or national guidance by searching
the Department of Health website www.dh.gov.uk. Here you can search for National Service
Frameworks, long-term conditions strategies, self-care strategies, public health issues, the
Expert Patient schemes and also access disease-specific libraries within the website.

Step 10: Activity 13.2.10

*The team approach: How is the patient looked after, by whom and how does it all join up
to enhance care?*

The team approach to patient care is very important. Identify all the health care and social
care professionals involved with looking after this group of patients. What is the role of each
professional? Is there any overlap, duplication of effort, omission of care, danger of different messages from different health care professionals? If so, how may this and the patient's
pharmaceutical care be improved?

Compare with good practice elsewhere. Is there a patient care pathway? If so, is this useful
or would implementing such be useful in the practice setting?

Constructing a new Therapeutic Framework for each new disease area you encounter, will help you to understand the way these medicines work and how the medicines interact with each other and across the lifespan. These related issues are all important to know when looking after your patient in any environment and clinical area. Activity 13.2 is designed to take you through this process step by step. Once mastered, you will have an excellent resource to help with your clinical practice now and in the future.

Conclusion

This chapter has introduced you to the concepts of pharmacology, pharmacokinetics and the evidence-based use of medicines. It has identified sources of information and guidance on where to look for practical information on medicines. By building a Therapeutic Framework you will be able to develop and deepen your knowledge. This introduction to medicines can be built on in practice and through further study. Medicines form an extremely important part of treatment. Therefore, it is vital that all members of the health care team are able to identify therapeutic and undesirable effects of medicines and support patients to gain the best possible outcome from drug treatment.

References

British National Formulary (BNF) (2008) Pharmaceutical Press, London.

Department of Health (DH) (2001) *National Service Framework for Diabetes*. DH, London, available at http://www.dh.gov.uk/en/Healthcare/NationalServiceFrameworks/Diabetes/DH_4015717

Medicines and Healthcare Products Regulatory Agency: Great Britain (n.d). *Medicines and Medical Devices: Regulation, What You Need to Know*, latest edn. HMSO, London, available at http://www.mhra.gov.uk/home/groups/comms-ic/documents/websiteresources/con2031677.pdf (accessed June 2008).

National Health Service/Prescription Pricing Division (NHS/PPD) (2008) *Update on Growth in Prescription Volume and Cost*. NHS Business Services Authority, available at http://www.ppa.org.uk/ppa/pres_vol_cost.htm

Nursing and Midwifery Council (NMC) (2007) *Essential Skills Clusters*. NMC Circular 07(2007) Annexe 2, NMC, London.

Rang H.P., Dale M.M., Ritter J.M. (2007) *Rang and Dale's Pharmacology*. Churchill Livingstone, Edinburgh.

Walker R., Whittlesea C. (2007) *Clinical Pharmacy and Therapeutics*. Churchill Livingstone, Edinburgh.

CHAPTER 14

Principles of Medicines Management

Linda Louise Childs

Introduction

This chapter identifies the supporting theory relating to the Essential Skills Clusters for medicines management (NMC 2007a). This will supplement your coursework, which along with your learned practice skills and your competence in drugs calculations will enable you to meet the required standards for registration in respect to medicines management. The nurse's role in medicines management across all health care sectors and relevant to all practice settings and groups including adult and the older person, mental health, learning disability and child within in-patient, primary care, schools and residential care is explored.

The specific learning outcomes addressed in this chapter link with the Nursing and Midwifery Council's (NMC 2007a) Essential Skills Clusters, and are identified below.

Learning outcomes

By the end of this chapter you will be able to do the following:

- Identify the nurses' role to enable you to work safely and effectively within the team regards medicines management.
- Identify legal, ethical and professional frameworks that underpin safe and effective medicines management.
- Understand the importance of partnerships with patients/clients to enable concordance when planning treatment.

What is a Medicine?

A medicine is any substance or combination of substances which may be administered for treating or preventing disease in human beings or animals, for making a medical diagnosis or for restoring, correcting or modifying physiological functions in human beings or animals (*Council Directive 65/65/ EEC*, EEC 1965).

The use of medicines is one strategy which, along with a number of therapeutic interventions, is widely employed in today's health care provision to maintain and promote heath and to prevent and treat illness. More than 2.5 million prescriptions are issued in England across community and hospital services each day (National Patient Safety Agency (NPSA) 2004). This represents significant activity and cost with each hospital in England and Wales administering 7000 medicine doses each day (Audit Commission 2001). Consequently, a large proportion of a nurses' time is spent managing medicines for their patients.

Definition of Medicines Management

In the context of the responsibility of the nurse, medicines management may be defined as the clinical, cost effective and safe use of medicines to ensure that the patients obtain the maximum benefit from the medicines they need, whilst minimising potential harm (DH 2004). Traditionally, doctors prescribed, pharmacists dispensed and nurses administered medicines. Today nurses and other health professionals are involved at all stages of the process, thus medicines management has become a multi-professional concern and nurses must work closely with all team members to ensure best patient care and outcomes.

Nurses' Role in Medicines Management

The nurse, in partnership with other members of the multidisciplinary team, is responsible for assessing, planning and implementing drug regimens, monitoring effects and educating patients regards their therapies. *Standards for Medicines Management* (NMC 2007b) set standards which all nurses must meet. Consequently, any nurse whose practice is in breach of these standards will be called to account and as a result of such a breach being upheld, may be deemed unfit to practice and have his or her name removed from the register and thus be unable to practice. Student nurses must therefore work towards attaining the medicines management proficiencies set within the Essential Skills Clusters (NMC 2007a) under the direct supervision of a registered nurse (usually their mentor).

The registered nurse is responsible for all delegated care delivered by the student, and both the nurse and student must confine their practice to activities within their scope of competence and adhere to local policy and guidelines. As the student nurse progresses and gains skills the supervision may become increasingly indirect to reflect the competence level achieved.

To safely administer medicines they should be given as ordered on the prescription and each nurse must

- be certain of the identity of the patient receiving the medicine;
- check that the patient is not allergic to the medication or that it is contraindicated;
- be aware of the patient's care plan;
- possess knowledge of the therapeutic use of the product, normal dosage, precautions, contraindications and side effects;
- establish the clarity of the prescription and/or the label on the medication to be dispensed (this must be legible and unambiguous);
- check that the product is within the expiry date;
- consider the dosage, weight where appropriate, method, route and timing of the administration in the context of the patient's condition, diagnoses and co-existing therapies;
- administer or withhold the medicine in the context of the patient's condition or where contraindications may manifest;
- contact the prescriber (or if unavailable another doctor or authorised prescriber) immediately if any contraindications or reactions, or where assessment of the patient indicates that the medicine is no longer suitable;
- make clear accurate legible and immediate record of all medicine administered, intentionally withheld or refused by the patient with the reason, and sign (follow any additional local guidelines);
- clearly countersign the signature of any student who has been supervised by the nurse in the administration of medicines. It is the nurse's responsibility to ensure that a record is made when delegating the administration of a medicine;
- witness that the medicine has been taken (not left to be taken later); and
- sign (a single signature is required); however, controlled drugs (CDs) given in secondary care/hospital settings require a second signature by the person witnessing the whole administration process including preparation and drawing up of injections.

Crushing medication. Tablets must never be crushed, capsules never broken unless advised by a pharmacist as this may alter their therapeutic properties or affect the rate at which the medicine is absorbed. If a patient has difficulty swallowing tablets, the prescriber must be notified so that a different preparation, for example liquid preparation, may be considered. The NMC advises against *disguising medication* by mixing in food or drink so that the patient is unaware that they are taking this. In exceptional circumstances a registered nurse who decides to disguise a medicine would need to be sure that this was in the patient's best interest and would remain accountable for all decisions and actions.

Substances for injection. These must not be prepared in advance of their immediate use nor may practitioners administer medication drawn into a syringe or container by another practitioner when not in their presence.

Patient-specific directions. These are the traditional and most common ways for any nurse to administer medicines, via a written instruction on a patient's record or ward drug chart, from a doctor, dentist, nurse or other prescriber, to a named patient.

Patient Group Directions

Patient Group Directions (PGDs) provide a legal framework for the supply and administration of medicine or vaccines directly to a patient, without the need for a prescription, subject to certain conditions being met. PGDs are for specified groups of patients and must be drawn up and signed by a doctor in advance of the treatment delivered by a registered nurse or certain qualified health professionals (DH 2000a). Since 2003, PGDs may be legally used in non-NHS organisations, independent hospital agencies and clinics registered under the *Care Standards Act* 2000, prison health care services, police services and defence medical services. Nurse training now requires nurses to have a knowledge of PGDs, although only registered nurses are permitted to administer a medicine under a PGD.

Employers normally initiate annual training and set and monitor standards for competence before registered nurses are sanctioned to supply and administer medicines by this method. The National Prescribing Centre (NPC 2004) provides a competency framework for staff using PGDs.

The competence required includes the ability to

- demonstrate knowledge of the condition presenting;
- demonstrate knowledge of the medication – actions and interactions, possible side effects, contraindications and how mechanisms may be altered, for example influence of age, renal conditions and so on;
- complete a holistic assessment;
- consider differential diagnoses;
- make a diagnoses;
- consider patient's perceptions;
- consider the non-pharmaceutical approaches;
- be aware of public health issues;
- offer health promotion; and
- work towards partnerships to enable concordance.

The supply of medicines under a PGD should be reserved for the limited number of cases where this offers an advantage to the patient without compromising safety (DH 2000a). Currently, PGDs are widely used in a number of health care settings: unscheduled and emergency care, walk-in centres and for the delivery of the childhood immunisation programme, flu vaccines and emergency contraception. Analgesics, including some CDs and antibiotics may now be administered under PGDs as they enable timely access to treatment and a reduction in waiting times. They must however only be used following a thorough assessment and diagnosis, with the patient's agreement, and nurses must select and implement the relevant PGD.

To comply with legislation each PGD must state the clinical condition, patient inclusion and exclusion criteria, information on the medicine, instructions for use, warnings, adverse reactions, arrangement for further advice, referral, follow-up and record keeping. Nurses proposing to use the PGD must be named by the Trust and a record kept (DH 2000a). The use of PGDs must also be consistent with appropriate professional relationships and accountability, with practitioners working within their scope of competence. Where treatment is long term or requires adjustment of dosage, PGDs are not considered suitable (Activity 14.1).

> **Activity 14.1**
>
> Why not explore this further with your mentor and learn more about PGDs. Access a variety of PGDs which may be adapted to meet specific needs from The NHS Electronic Library for Health at http://www.library.nhs.uk/emergency/SearchResults.aspx?tabID=288&catID=7055

Caution is required when prescribing or developing PGDs for antimicrobials, black triangle drugs, those used 'off label' or for children. For antimicrobials, consideration of the risks of increasing resistance within the general community is a priority (DH 2003; BMA 2006), and advice from a microbiologist and the drugs and therapeutics committee must be upheld. 'Off label' refers to drugs used outside their summary of product characteristics, often used for children, their use should be the exception and justified by best practice.

Homely Remedies

Homely remedies involve the administration of Pharmacy Only Medicines (POM) and General Sales List Medicines available over the counter. These may be administered by named nurses under a local protocol drawn up by a doctor or pharmacist which states the condition to treat, the indications, dose and dose frequency. Time limit for the length of time to treat before referring to a doctor must be stated.

Today's health care requires nurses to extend their knowledge and skills to deliver complete episodes of care (DH 2000b, 2006). Nurse prescribing is identified as an essential skill to enable autonomous practice to meet patient's needs for timely access to medicines.

The Medicinal Product: *Prescription by Nurses Act* (1992)

This Act enabled experienced nurses to undertake further training in preparation to meet the standards set for recording nurse prescribing status on the NMC register. Prescriptive authority has been extended, and there are now two categories of nurse prescriber (see Box 14.1 for categories).

Administering Medicines

Observing the six Rights provides an easy-to-remember checklist for consideration prior to administration:

- The Right Medication
- The Right Amount
- The Right Time
- The Right Patient
- The Right Route
- Right Record to record administration.

BOX 14.1

Categories of Nurse Prescriber. Reproduced under the terms of the Click-Use Licence

(V100) and (V150) Nurse Independent Prescriber

Those undertaking a Community Specialist Practice/Public Health programme may achieve training for recording V100 nurse prescriber status to prescribe from the limited formulary (BMA/CPHVA/RCN 2007).

New programmes (NMC 2007c) enable experienced first-level nurses without a community qualification to complete training for recording V150 nurse prescriber status to prescribe from the limited formulary.

(V300) Independent and Supplementary Nurse Prescriber

From May 2006 Nurse Independent & Supplementary Prescribers may train to achieve V300 recorded entry on the NMC register to independently prescribe any licensed medicine listed within the *British National Formulary* (BNF) and some CDs (this may be expanded in the future) or prescribe any licensed medicine as a Supplementary Prescriber.

Supplementary Prescribing is initiated from an existing Clinical Management Plan to which the patient has agreed, and which has been set up in advance of the nurse prescribing. It documents the partnership between the doctor as independent prescriber and the nurse as supplementary prescriber and indicates the medication which may be prescribed (DH 2005).

Nurses have an important role to play in educating patients to competently manage their medicines and adhere to their treatment regimens. Whilst patients remain in hospital, their adherence to prescribed medications regimes is monitored and recorded. However, evidence indicates high rates of non-adherence to medicines regimes following discharge from hospital (Horner *et al.* 2005). Educating patients about their medication regime increases their knowledge and understanding of the importance of adhering to their treatment. Planned self-administration programmes implemented before discharge promote adherence and patient understanding (Deeks & Byatt 2000). The nurse must be satisfied that the individual is capable of safe administration.

Compliance aids may be used to assist patients to adhere to their regime. Dosing aids may be prepared in advance to hold the dispensed medicines for each dosage on a daily basis for one week. Nurses must assess the patient's suitability and ability to use the chosen compliance aid safely. Filling a compliance aid entails *repackaging dispensed medicines*; this is usually done by agreement of the pharmacy team. A risk assessment is required regards the potential for error and the possibility that the properties of the drug may alter as a result of re-packaging and thus may not be covered by product licence. Re-packaging should only be carried out with agreement from both the dispensing pharmacist, and employer and should be covered by local policy/Standard Operating Procedure.

Self-administration of Medicines and Administration by Carers

Many hospital and residential settings enable self-administration of medicines. Nurses retain a duty of care relating to this activity and also to the use of patients'

BOX 14.2

Self-administration assessment levels

Level 1

The nurse remains responsible for the safe storage of the medicines and supervises the administration process ensuring that the patient has an understanding of the purpose and actions of the medicine.

Level 2

The nurse is responsible for the safe storage of the medicine. The patient asks the nurse to open the medicine cabinet/locker at the time the medicines are due. The patient self-administers the medicine under the supervision of the nurse.

Level 3

The patient accepts full responsibility for the storage and administration of the medicines. The nurse checks the patient's suitability and compliance on a regular basis using local policy to determine that they remain capable of safe administration and this is recorded.

Nurses have continuing responsibility for recognising and acting upon changes in a patient's condition regarding the safety of the patient and others. If a patient withholds consent to self-administer and other arrangements are made, information about their medicines and what to do following discharge must still be given (NMC 2007b).

---

own medications. Where self/carer administration of medicines has been agreed, the following points should be considered:

- Patients/carers share the responsibility for their actions relating to administration of medicines.
- Patients/carers can withdraw consent at any time.

The following information should be provided before commencing self-administration:

- the name of the medicine;
- why they are taking it;
- dose and frequency;
- actions and common side effects and what to do if they occur;
- any special instructions;
- duration of the course or how to obtain further supplies.

The pharmacy will supply medicines fully labelled, with directions for use.

The NMC (2007b) recommends that patients be assessed for suitability on three levels and the level determined is recorded (Box 14.2).

Patients who may be confused must not be given custody of their medicines but may self-administer on levels one and two only. In the hospital setting, this includes patients under the influence of anaesthetic agents or those acutely ill who may at times be confused. Reassessment at a later stage may determine suitability to self-administer.

The above also applies to *Patients with a past history of drug or alcohol misuse* who may require extra education, supervision and reinforcement in self-administration of their medicines (NMC 2007b). Local policies using the NMC guidance for self-administration of medicinal products reflect best practice (Activity 14.2).

Section 5

Activity 14.2

With your mentor discuss local and national medicines management guidance.
Ask your mentor to assist you to locate medicines management policy/guidelines relating to
   your practice area and familiarise yourself with these.
Identify your guidelines for medicines management within your education institute.

Concordance, Compliance and Adherence

Concordance is the term widely used for the partnership approach in reaching agreement between health care practitioner and a patient as regards the prescribing and taking of medicines according to the recommended therapeutic regime.

Compliance and adherence are terms which refer to the intended outcomes of medicines taking. When a patient, for whatever reason, does not adhere to the prescribed medication regime either deliberately or unintentionally, this action is referred to as non-compliance. Cultural and religious beliefs, past experiences and individual health beliefs may influence an individual's views about the benefits of taking medicines (Horner *et al.* 2005). It is important that patients' beliefs and preferences are explored (Haynes *et al.* 2002) and any concurrent treatments identified before initiating a new treatment. It is estimated that as many as 50% of those with long-term conditions are non-compliant with their prescribed medications regime (Healthcare Commission 2007). Levels of non-concordance are significantly higher for those where the effects of their medications regime impact on their behaviour and lifestyle (Haynes *et al.* 2002; WHO 2003). The elderly, those with mental health conditions and those with learning disabilities have been found to have a significant incidence of non-adherence. The Healthcare Commission (2007) suggests that non-compliance may be due to the following:

- Conflict with cultural values and personal wishes
- Problems with access (collecting prescription, cost, opening bottle)
- Cognitive ability – forgetfulness
- Concerns about effects/side effects (either through understanding or misunderstanding)
- Inadequate education on how medicines should be taken
- Lack of information about condition and treatment
- Incompatible with life style.

Reasons for non-compliance are complex and, although no single approach appears more effective in achieving concordance, there is consensus that some useful strategies to promote concordance are the following:

- a partnership approach which considers a patient's culture, health beliefs and preferences;
- employing educational strategies using verbal and written information to reinforce instructions;
- clear labelling of product displaying dosage and frequency;

- selecting the simplest regime, for example prescribing once daily doses where possible;
- reviewing the patients' understanding and encouraging questions;
- gaining carer/family support where appropriate.

Formal and informal opportunities to review a person's medication regime may be usefully employed by practitioners. By asking which medication is taken in what quantity by which route and how frequently, nurses may assess adherence to the prescribed regime, address any issues and give advice to facilitate concordance. Strategies to build partnerships between service users and health and social care practitioners are promoted (DH 2008a) to facilitate safe use of medicines to enable best therapeutic outcomes.

In addition to prescription medicines, individuals may also receive *alternative* and *complementary therapies* or be self treating: taking, vitamin or food supplements, herbal, homeopathic or *over the counter medication*. Many of these treatments and therapies have no robust evidence to support their effectiveness, although there may be a commonly held perception that whilst their effectiveness is unproven, they will do no harm. This may not be the case, as there is evidence that serious inter-actions may occur when certain products or some foods are consumed with some prescribed medication. This also applies to the effects of *smoking, caffeine, alcohol* and *street drugs*. Although the NMC advises that only nurses with additional training and competence should administer complimentary medicine/alternative remedies, all nurses should alert the prescriber of the potential for interactions (see BNF, Appendix 1, BMA 2008a) and advise the patient accordingly. Baseline infor-mation on the safety of medicines, storage and lifestyle advice should be accessed by all patients. Information leaflets offer a useful resource to reinforce this.

Medicines and Vulnerable People

Administering and/or prescribing medications for children. The NMC (2006) advises that issuing medicines under a PGD for a child is confined to nurses with relevant knowledge, competence and experience. Nurses must work within their competence and refer to another practitioner competent in that particular field when care falls beyond their expertise and competence. Attention to the child's weight, size and maturity when considering suitability of the medicine is imper-ative (see *British National Formulary for Children*, BMA 2008b) and care is needed with calculating and preparing doses (WHO 2007). NPSA (2007) reports that of all reported medications, errors more than 10% occur in children under 4 years old. Guidance within the National Service Framework (NSF) for children (*Medicines for Children and Young People*, DH/DfES 2004) should be adhered to and consideration given to the prior establishment of a trusting relationship with the child. Adequate time should be allowed to prepare and comfort the child and assistance from a parent or other team member may be required. Play may be used to prepare the child for the administration of the medication and the child may be empowered to choose whether the parent or nurse administer. Be truthful regarding painful procedures such as injections; adopt a calm, confident, kind but firm approach and always reward the child with positive feedback. Administration should be timely according to prescribed regime and may differ significantly from that for an adult (see Chapter 13). Failing to administer medicines on time is an issue particularly where a child is nursed on a general ward rather than a children's ward (NPSA 2007). For *children with complex needs* a competent other/parent (as assessed by the nurse) may administer medicines to a named child providing that an individual care plan has been written and signed off by the registered nurse. This is often employed in community and palliative care settings.

Administering and/or prescribing medications for patients/clients with learning disabilities. The nurse should determine the patients' understanding and choice when considering consent, and act in the patients' best interest at all times. The nurse may adapt a relevant approach to develop a therapeutic relationship to strive to gauge the client's/patient's understanding of the significance of administering the medication. Consideration of physical conditions, mental heath and abilities will help the prescriber determine the most suitable route and preparation for the prescribed drug. There is a high incidence of physical and mental illness which remains undetected and thus untreated within this group of patients. Nurses have an advocacy role to facilitate diagnoses and appropriate treatment of any co-existing conditions and minor ailments.

Administering and/or prescribing medications for patients/clients in mental health settings. Challenges with achieving adherence with drug regimes are a particular issue in mental health settings (Healthcare Commission 2007) with consideration of mental capacity and consent key issues. However, in circumstances where the patient has been detained for appropriate treatment subject to the *Mental Health Act*, administration of medication, which contravenes the patient's expressed wishes, is lawfully upheld for a stated period of time. Although it is recognised that considerable steps are taken to establish concordance with patients by those working in Mental Health Trusts, a ward-level audit, undertaken by pharmacists, identified that 46% of those reviewed had issues with adherence compared to 12% in general settings (Hull & East Yorkshire CMT 2007). Some medication regimes such as antipsychotic therapy require close monitoring to ensure that the benefits of the medications given outweigh the risks. Patient preference and carer perspectives must be considered when planning all care (NPSA 2006b).

Nice Guidance, national and local policy should be observed. The Prescribing Observatory for Mental Health (POMH–UK) was set up in 2005 to maintain standards for prescribed medications and it provides useful information for best practice. Where it is known that the patient's evolving condition, treatment or prescribed medications may impede thinking, a patient's decision on care should be explored as early as possible and prior to starting the treatment if possible. An advance directive stating what treatments and medications the patient would wish to engage should they lack the capacity at a later date either temporarily or permanently is recommended (Healthcare Commission 2007).

Influences on Decision-making

When considering our actions we are bound by NMC codes, standards and guidelines, for students guidelines set by their training institution by local standards and guidelines within the clinical practice area and by the laws of the country. Best evidence, NSFs and guidelines, for example NICE, also guide our practice and decision-making. Ethics may be engaged to guide decision, by enabling wider consideration of the issues pertaining to a particular challenge or intervention.

The ethics of medicines management

Beauchamp and Childress (2001) propose four ethical principles:

- Respect for autonomy
- Benefice
- Non-maleficence
- Justice

which may be supplemented by the following four rules:

- Veracity – truth telling
- Privacy
- Confidentiality
- Fidelity – trustworthiness.

These principles and rules have been employed within the NMC (2008) code to enable us to consider options to make sense of conflicting view points and provide patient-centred care which may be applied to medicines management (see Chapter 9 for more information).

Respect for autonomy. A patient's choice of preference for treatment or whether to decline treatment is protected by the law. The nurse has a duty to protect and support the health of individual patients, clients and the wider benefits of society. However, this may, in some cases, raise ethical dilemmas. A patient with a sore throat may request an antibiotic believing that this is best; however, the prescriber's decision to withhold treatment, in line with present guidance for the rational prescribing of antimicrobials to prevent proliferation of resistant strains of bacteria which pose a threat to the wider population, promotes the greater good for society.

Beneficence to do good, to act for the well-being of the individual. Nurses must enable patients to adhere to their prescribed drugs regime in order to obtain optimal benefit from their treatment. From a legal perspective nurses have a duty to make available services and treatments to benefit patients.

Non-maleficence. Nurses are required to safeguard the patient/client from harm. This is also a legal requirement. An awareness of the actions, interactions, contraindications, and side effects of medications enable the nurse to monitor effects of medications and take steps to reduce the potential for harm.

Negligence. This is failure to provide adequate care to guard against harm. This may occur through administering a medication which is contraindicated, or by omitting to give medication as prescribed or by failure to administer a dose of an anti-epileptic drug to a patient on time resulting in the patient having a seizure.

Accountability. Nurses are accountable for their practice to their patients, employer, their professional body – NMC and to the law. Nurses must work within their level of competence and adhere to the *Standards for Medicines Management* (NMC 2007b). The standard of care expected from a nurse prescriber would be expected to exceed that of a first level competent nurse thus reflecting variance in levels of accountability. Accordingly, the NMC (2006) has set *Standards of Proficiency for Nurse and Midwife Prescribers*.

The law and medicines management

Civil law is concerned with proceedings which fall outside the criminal law. These include employment law, breach of contract and so on, and Tort which includes damages resulting from negligence. Nurses' medicines management activity must remain at all times within the terms of their employment and remain in accordance with their job specification, local guidelines, protocols and policy, in order that their employer carries vicarious liability.

Criminal law relates to crimes against the state such as damage to property or deliberate harm perpetrated on others. Those found guilty of such actions may face a custodial sentence. Examples include the cases of the former nurse Beverley Alitt (DH 1994) and Dr Harold Shipman, both were charged and sentenced under the criminal law for wilfully causing death by administering lethal doses of drugs to patients in their care. Following the resulting Shipman inquiry (Smith 2004) clinical governance structures were reviewed and recommendations to protect the public and prevent recurrence were implemented.

Justice implies equality in accessing health care services or treatments available. Evolving health care technology along with increased demand for treatments and rising costs of medicines has not been met with proportionate increases in funding. This resulted in a rationing of health care with waiting lists for treatments and a post code lottery, whereby patients living within one area are able to access a particular treatment funded by the NHS when the same treatment is unavailable to those living in another postcode area. Consequently, a rationalisation of treatments has been adopted both locally and nationally to enable the best outcomes. The implementation of local cost-effective formularies and medicines-review initiatives have reduced individual treatment costs enabling higher numbers to be treated effectively within the health care budget. The implementation of NSFs (see NSFs 2006) and NICE guidance have provided an agreed national baseline to enable equity in access to treatments funded by the NHS (Activity 14.3).

Activity 14.3

Access the NICE Guidance for Chronic Obstructive Airways Disease (COPD) at http://www. nice.nhs.uk/guidance/index.jsp?action=byID&o=10938. What treatment and medication are recommended?

Reflect on the nursing care you have been involved within practice or select a condition which you are interested in. Can you identify a NSF or NICE guidance to identify best practice?

Consent is always required before medicines are administered and with *informed consent* nurses must give clear information about treatment planned. Thus nurses require a knowledge of illness trajectories, pharmacology and therapeutics to provide information, regarding treatment options and possible outcomes to enable patients to make an informed decision as regards proposed treatment options. Section on Consent in Chapter 9 of this book contains more on this important subject.

Legislative controls and medicines management

Medicines have the potential to benefit health but may also cause harm; consequently, legislative controls are in place for the manufacture, distribution, sale, storage, labelling and administration of drugs which provide frameworks for practice and protect patients from harm.

Medicines are classified under the *Medicines Act 1968* as the following:

General Sales List Medicines (GSL) – sold without supervision.
Pharmacy only Medicines (P) – sold under the supervision of a pharmacist.
Prescription only Medicine (POM) – sold or supplied in accordance with a
    prescription produced by an authorised prescriber.

Prescriptions must be legible, completed in indelible ink, signed and dated by the prescriber, accurately provide the patient's identity, specify medicine, form dose and dose frequency, and minimal dose interval. For all requirements see BNF (BMA 2008a).

Other key legislations which control the use and handling of medicines include the following:
   The POM and Human Use Order (1997) enables nurses to administer medicines generally, under prescription and in accordance with PGDs.
   The Misuse of Drugs Act 1971 controls the use, manufacture, supply and possession of certain drugs to prevent misuse of CDs, which are believed to have potential for abuse/addiction and are classified according to their harmfulness when misused as classes A the most harmful, B and C. Penalties applicable to offences involving CDs are apportioned according to this classification.
   The Misuse of Drugs Regulations 2001 classifies drugs as schedules 1–5 with the most stringent controls for schedules 1 and 2 with lesser controls for 3, 4 and 5. It is unlawful to possess and supply CDs in schedule 1 unless specified in a professional capacity within this act. Any person identified with an addiction to CDs (such as cocaine, methadone, morphine, diamorphine, amphetamines and pethadine) must be reported by the doctor to the Regional or National Drugs Misuse Database/Centre as noted in the BNF.
   The Misuse of Drugs Act (Supply to Addicts) Regulations 1997 require that only doctors licensed by the Home Secretary may prescribe, administer and supply diamorphine, dipipanone and cocaine in the treatment of addiction. However, other prescribers may prescribe these drugs for patients (including addicts) for treating pain from organic disease or trauma.

Section 5

Controlled Drugs (Supervision of Management and Use) Regulations 2006, the key provisions are the following:

- All health care organisations and independent hospitals are required to appoint an accountable officer to implement set standards for the management of CDs.
- A duty of collaboration for health care organisations and local and national agencies including professional regulatory bodies, police forces, the Healthcare Commission and the Commission for Social Care Inspection, to share intelligence on CD issues.
- A power of entry and inspection for the police and other nominated people to enter premises to inspect stocks and records of CDs.

Safe Custody of CDs apply to schedule 1, 2 and some schedule 3. All must be locked in a metal cabinet/cupboard which is fixed to the wall or floor with bolts which are inaccessible from outside the cabinet.

- The cupboard must be dedicated to the storage of CDs. No other medicines or items may be stored in the CD cupboard.
- CDs must be locked in cupboard when not in use.
- Stock will be regularly checked recorded and signed.

Key-holding and access to CDs

- The Registrant in Charge is responsible for the CD key
- Key-holding may be delegated to other suitably trained members of staff but the legal responsibility rests with the Registrant in Charge.

Administration of CDs

- These should be administered in line with relevant legislation and local standard interest of patient care (and adhere to the standard procedures for administration of medicines) (see guidance DH 2008b).
- A second nurse should witness and check the order, preparation and administration of the medicine, and the safe disposal of any excess – for example in the case of an injection requiring half an ampoule to be given as ordered the remaining drug should be immediately disposed of according to local guidance/standard operating procedures.
- Stock balance should be carried out and recorded.
- The CD should be given immediately by the nurse (or personally supervised if delegated to a student).
- This should be recorded as per standard procedure, be signed and dated by both nurses. Where this is not possible a second person who has been assessed as competent may witness the whole administration process and sign the record.

Substance misuse settings – In cases of direct patient administration of oral medication from stock, the nurse is required to administer the dose and personally supervise and witness the immediate ingestion of prescribed medication for example methadone. The whole process must be witnessed, recorded/signed for by the nurse and a second nurse or person assessed as competent.

Misuse of Drugs Regulations and the Health Act (2006) introduced changes affecting the prescribing, record keeping and destruction of CDs. This requires

---

Activity 14.4

Read the DH Guidance and Policy Re Controlled Drugs by visiting the DH webpage http://
www.dh.gov.uk/en/Policyandguidance/Medicinespharmacyandindustry/Prescriptions/
ControlledDrugs/index.htm

---

new regulations to be instated relating to governance and monitoring of CDs,
including directives for the requisition, receipt, transporting and stock checking. New regulations (DH 2008b) governing the record keeping for CDs came
into force in January 2008 for recording: when CDs are obtained, when CDs are
supplied in response to prescription and the disposal/destruction of CDs (for
further guidance see NMC 2007b) (Activity 14.4).

Safety and Governance Structures

The prescriber is required to assess whether the known benefits of taking a medicine outweigh the risk posed by possible side effects and make a decision based on
best predicted outcome. Medicines are used frequently in health care, consequently
the potential for risk, which is inherent in all aspects of health care delivery, is
high, with the outcome that some patients are harmed as a result of taking their
medicines. When medicines have caused harm but no error took place, the incident
is judged to be non-preventable and is referred to as an Adverse Drug Reaction.

Adverse Drug Reaction (ADR). An example is a patient who develops an allergy
to an antibiotic taken for the first time, which could not have been predicted.
All drugs reactions are required to be notified to the Medicines and Healthcare
Products Regulatory Agency/Commission of Human Medicines by completing a
yellow card; see Chapter 13.

Errors with the use of medicines. These are the most common threat to patient
safety (Neale *et al.* 2001) and pose concern worldwide. An 'error' is described as a
planned action which fails to achieve the desired outcome. Medications errors may
occur at any stage of the medicines process (Figure 14.1).
   An example of a preventable incident is a patient with a known allergy to penicillin who is prescribed a penicillin medicine and develops an allergic reaction as
a consequence. All causes of harm and potential harm including drug prescribing
and administration errors must be reported via local risk management systems.
So must 'near misses' or 'no harm' events. A drug error that was noticed before
the drug was administered is an example of a near miss. An example of a no
harm error is a patient given 500 mg of flucloxacillin when prescribed 250 mg. On
detecting errors or ADRs nurses must take immediate action to protect the patient
from potential harm and report as soon as possible to the prescriber and manager/
employer (according to local policy) and document the event and actions taken.

The National Patient Safety Agency (NPSA). NPSA was established in 2001
to improve patient safety by promoting a culture of reporting and learning

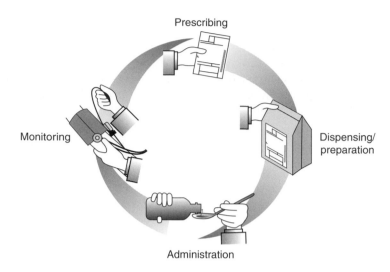

Figure 14.1   The medication process. Source: From NPSA (2007), *Safety in Doses*. Reproduced under the terms of the Click-Use Licence.

from adverse incidents and near misses. Organisations are required to inform the NPSA of locally reported patient safety issues. Staff may anonymously report incidents in which they are involved or witness directly to the NPSA (www.npsa.nhs.uk/staffeform/).The National Reporting and Learning System (NRLS) analyses this information, publishes statistics, identifies trends and delivers effective, practical and timely solutions. Improving safety requires staff to acknowledge and learn from mistakes (NPSA 2004, 2006a). For this a change in both the culture and systems in the workplace was called for (DH 2000c) to develop an open learning environment, to challenge poor practice, report any actions which may cause harm and learn from mistakes and near misses. Nurses have embraced these principles and reflected the desired cultural shift in reporting errors more so than other practitioners (DH 2007). Roberts *et al.* (2002) identified that nurses reported 45% of all recorded errors. Although medicines incidents and near misses are believed to remain under-reported training for health professionals has embraced the importance of this cultural shift and it is hoped that by reporting, and learning from events, and developing frameworks for scrutiny, medicines safety will be enhanced (NPSA 2004, 2006a).

Incidents reported, either directly or through the employer, enable the NPSA to map events and causal factors. It is more important to identify why and how a safety incident occurred, to learn from this to prevent recurrence rather than to attribute blame to one person (NPSA 2006a). NHS organisations are informed of recommendations from national inquiries, and alerts are circulated in order to take steps to prevent similar safety incidents. Focus is given to the conditions under which practitioners work and how these may predispose errors. It is only by acknowledging these predisposing conditions that system defences may be developed to avoid recurrence.

Medicines safety incidents

The multidisciplinary team should analyse the patient safety incident and review documentation and records when conducting incident analysis. Guidelines and training on analysis of incidents such as root cause analysis and appropriate interventions are provided on the NPSA website with a choice of 11 tools to consider contributory factors NPSA (2004).

Patient feedback is an important part of risk identification and risk management. Being open decreases the trauma felt by patients following a patient safety incident (Vincent & Coulter 2002). The NPSA (2005a) provides guidance for developing a consistent approach to handling communications following a patient safety incident resulting in harm. The NPSA (2005b) recommends that a senior practitioner with good communication skills empathetically leads an open and honest discussion with the patient and his or her significant others with support by either the risk manager or clinical lead. Focus should centre on clear explanations and the patient's or significant other's agenda whilst seeking resolution.

Nurses have a responsibility to monitor and audit all care including medicines management in order to maintain safe and high-quality care at all times (NMC 2008). Many patients receive care from both the acute and primary care sector and it is following discharge from acute care that patients are most at risk of medication errors. The Royal Pharmaceutical Society (RPSGB 2006) found 20% of patients experience an adverse event following discharge from acute care or between care providers. Further issues identified were that 25% of discharge letters were lost in the post and that 80% of consultant's letters took more than a month to reach the GP. The World Health Organisation (2007) published guidance on assuring medication accuracy at transition in care from one setting to another. The NPSA (2007) cite 7070 reported incidents of medications errors at admission and discharge of adults to health care settings between November 2003 and March 2007. Of these 30 resulted in severe harm and 2 were fatal. To address these issues NPSA/NICE (2007) set guidance for best practice, recommending a two-stage procedure. Stage 1: That a comprehensive record of current medication is made within 24 hours of admission, any discrepancies, changes, deletions and additions should be noted. Stage 2: Full reconciliation, compares the list at stage 1 with the information most recently available through identifying and resolving discrepancies in relation to the patient's diagnosis and care plan and accurately recording outcome.

Recommendations are for the pharmacists and the wider team to prioritise accurate recording of medication and alert the patient's physician of any new or changed medication. The advantages of the imminent introduction of the *electronic patient medical record* have the potential to improve the situation by providing an accessible summary of the individual's medications. *Electronic prescriptions* have the potential to increase safety by recording prescribed and dispensed medicines and by providing alerts specific to a patient's care regards risk, reactions and interactions (NHS 2006, *Connecting for Health*).

Conclusion

This chapter has explored the nurse's role in medicines management and identified some supporting theory to underpin the Essential Skills Clusters for medicines

---

Activity 14.5

Further reading and resources

Galbraith A., Bullock S., Menias E., Hunt B., Richards A., (2007) *Fundamentals of Pharmacology an Applied Approach for Nursing and Health,* 2nd edn. Pearson, England.
NMC (2007) *Standards for Medicines Management.* NMC, London, available at http://www.nmc-uk.org/aFrameDisplay.aspx?DocumentID=3732

---

management (NMC 2007a). By developing an understanding of evidence, frameworks and principles, you will build a foundation on which to expand your practice to meet the needs of your patients/clients and the proficiencies for entry to the NMC register. Activity 14.5 provides futher resources to anchor essential medicines management knowledge.

References

Audit Commission (2001) *A Spoonful of Sugar: Medicines Management in NHS Hospitals.* HMSO, London.

Beauchamp T.L., Childress T.F. (2001) *Principles of Biomedical Ethics*, 5th edn. Oxford University Press, Oxford.

British Medical Association (BMA) (2006) *Healthcare Associated Infections: Strategies for Improvement.* Improving Health, available at www.bma.org.optimaluseofantimicrobials

British Medical Association (BMA) (2008a) *British National Formulary.* RSPGB/BMA, London, available at www.bnf.org

British Medical Association (BMA) (2008b) *British National Formulary for Children.* RPS/BMJ, London, available at www.bnfc.org

British Medical Association/CPHVA/RCN (2007) *Nurse Prescribers' Formulary for Community Practitioners: NPF 2007–2009.* BMJ/RPS, London, available at www.bnfc.org

Deeks P.A., Byatt K. (2000) Are patients who self administer their medicines in hospital more satisfied with their care? *Journal of Advanced Nursing* 31(2): 395–400.

Department of Health (DH) (1994) *The Allitt Inquiry.* Clothier C. (chair). HMSO, London.

Department of Health (DH) (2000a) *HSC Patient Group Directions in England.* DH, London. 2000/026 (on line) 2/3/08, available at http://www.dh.gov.uk/assetRoot/04/01/22/60/04012260.pdf

Department of Health (DH) (2000b) *The NHS Plan.* HMSO, London.

Department of Health (DH) (2000c) *An Organisation with Memory: Learning from an Expert Group from Adverse Events.* HMSO, London.

Department of Health (DH) (2003) *Winning Ways: Working Together to Reduce Health Care Associated Infections in England.* DH, London.

Department of Health (DH) (2004) *Building a Safer NHS for Patients: Improving Medication Safety.* DH, London.

Department of Health (DH) (2005) *Supplementary Prescribing by Nurses, Pharmacists, Physiotherapists, Chiropodists, Podiatrists and Radiographers within the NHS in England: A Guide for Implementation.* DH, London.

Department of Health (DH) (2006) *Improving Patients Access to Medicines. A Guide to Implementing Nurse and Pharmacist Prescribing within the NHS in England.* DH, London.

Department of Health (DH) (2007) *Guidance on the Management of Safe Use of Controlled Drugs in Secondary Care in England: Controlled Drugs in Acute Care.* DH, London.

Department of Health (DH) (2008a) *Medicines Management Everybody's Business. A Guide for Service Users, Carers and Social Care Practitioners. New Ways of Working in Mental Health.* NIMHE National Workforce Programme, London.

Department of Health (DH) (2008b) *Safer Management of Controlled Drugs: Changes to Record Keeping Requirements Guidance (for England only).* Department of Health, London.

Department of Health/Department for Education & Skills (DH/DfES) (2004) *Medicines for Children and Young People.* DH, London, available at http://www.dh.gov.uk/en/Publicationsandstatistics/Publications/PublicationsPolicyAndGuidance/Browsable/DH_4117980

European Economic Community (EEC) (1965) *Council Directive 65/65/EEC, Medicinal Products.* European Economic Union, Brussels.

Haynes R.B., McDonald H.P., Garg A.X., Montague P. (2002) *Interactions for Helping Patients Follow Prescriptions for Medications.* Cochrane Review 2: 2002, Oxford.

Healthcare Commission (2007) *Talking about Medicines. The Management of Medicines in Trusts providing Mental Health Services.* Healthcare Commission, London.

Horner R., Weinman J., Barber N., Elliot R., Morgan M. (2005) *Concordance, Adherence and Compliance in Medicines Taking.* Report for the National Co-ordinating Centre for the NHS Service Delivery Organisation. NCCSDO, London.

Hull & East Yorkshire CMT (2007) *Involving Patients Best Practice in Talking about Medicines,* Healthcare Commission, p. 16.

The Medicinal Product: *Prescription by Nurses Act etc.* (1992) Chapter 28. HMSO, London, available at http://www.opsi.gov.uk/acts/acts1992/ukpga_19920028_en_1.htm

National Health Service (NHS) (2006) *Connecting for Health: Electronic Care Records and Prescribing. Connecting For Health Clinical Collection.* Issue 2 Autumn 2006. NHS, London.

The National Prescribing Centre (NPC) (2004) *Patient Group Directions. A Practical Guide and Framework of Competencies for all Professionals using PGDs.* NPC, Liverpool, available at npc.co.uk/publications/pgd/outline-framework.doc

National Patient Safety Agency (NPSA) (2004) *Seven Steps to Patient Safety.* NPSA, London.

National Patient Safety Agency (NPSA) (2005a) *Being Open: Communicating Patient Safety Incidents with Patients and Their Carers.* NPSA, London.

National Patient Safety Agency (NPSA) (2005b) *Being Open When Patients are Harmed.* NPSA, London.

National Patient Safety Agency (NPSA) (2006a) *Seven Steps to Patient Safety for Primary Care.* NPSA, London.

National Patient Safety Agency (NPSA) (2006b) *With Safety in Mind: Mental Health Services and Patient Safety.* NPSA, London.

National Patient Safety Agency (NPSA) (2007) *Safety in Doses: Medications Safety Incidents in the NHS,* 4th Report. NPSA, London, available at http://www.npsa.nhs.uk/site/media/documents/2755_PSO_Medicines.pdf

National Patient Safety Agency (NPSA)/NICE (2007) *Technical Patient Safety Solutions for Medicines Reconciliation on Admission of Adults to Hospital.* NPSA/NICE, London.

National Service Frameworks (NSFs) (2006) *National Service Frameworks in England NHS.* Home page http://www.nhs.uk/NSF/Pages/Nationalserviceframeworks.aspx

Neale G., Woloshynowych M., Vincent C. (2001) Exploring the causes of adverse events in NHS hospital practice. *Journal of Research in Social Medicine* 94: 322–330.

Nursing and Midwifery Council (NMC) (2006) *Standards of Proficiency for Nurse and Midwife Prescribers.* NMC, London.

Nursing and Midwifery Council (NMC) (2007a) *Essential Skills Clusters*. NMC Circular 07 (2007), Annexe 2, NMC, London.

Nursing and Midwifery Council (NMC) (2007b) *Standards for Medicines Management*. NMC, London, available at www.nmc-uk.org

Nursing and Midwifery Council (NMC) (2007c) *Standards of Educational Preparation for Prescribing from the Community Nurse Prescribers Formulary for Nurses without a Specialist Practitioner Qualification – V150*. NMC Circular 2006/7 (December 2007), NMC, London.

Nursing and Midwifery Council (NMC) (2008) *The Code: Standards of Conduct, Performance and Ethics for Nurses and Midwives*. NMC, London.

Roberts D.E., Spencer M.G., Burfield R., Bowden S. (2002) An analysis of dispensing errors in UK hospitals. *International Journal of Pharmacology Practice* 10: R6 (supplement).

Royal Pharmaceutical Society (RPSGB) (2006) *Moving Patient's Medicines Safely: Discharge and Transfer Planning Book*. RSPGB, London.

Smith J. (2004) *The Shipman Inquiry 4th Report Regulations of Controlled drugs*. TSO, Norwich, available at http://www.the-shipman-inquiry.org.uk/fourthreport.asp

Vincent C.A., Coulter A. (2002) Patient safety: what about the patient? *Quality and Safety in Health Care* 11(1): 76–80.

World Health Organisation (WHO) (2003) *Adherence to Long Term Therapies: Evidence for Action*. WHO, Geneva.

World Health Organisation (WHO) (2007) *Promoting Safety of Medicines for Children*. WHO, Geneva, available at http://www.who.int/medicines/publications/essentialmedicines/Promotion_safe_med_childrens.pdf

Additional Cited Drugs Legislation

The Misuse of Drugs Regulations (2001) *Dangerous Drugs*. Statutory Instrument 3998 2001. HMSO, London.

The Misuse of Drugs Act (Supply to addicts) Regulations (1997) TSO, London, available at http://drugs.homeoffice.gov.uk/publication-search/drug-licences/General_Licence_to_Practiti1.pdf

Controlled Drugs (Supervision of Management and Use) Regulations (2006) Statutory Instrument 2006 No. 3148. TSO, London.

Misuse of Drugs Regulations and the Health Act (2006) Statutory Instrument 2006 No. 1450. TSO, London.

Index